# ICD-10-CM Coding Guidelines

# Made Easy

# 2017

## Terry Tropin, MSHAI, RHIA, CCS-P

## AHIMA-Approved ICD-10-CM/PCS Trainer

# Reviewers

Corinne M. Smith, MBA, RHIA, CCS, CDIP, CHDA
Professor, Program Coordinator
Health Information Management Program
Montgomery College, Maryland

Tasha E. Green, MS, RHIA, CHTS-TR
AHIMA Certified ICD-10 Trainer
Program Director and Associate Professor
Health Information Management Department
Prince George's Community College

Lauren Pitts, RHIT, CCS, CCS-P
Sibley Memorial Hospital
Washington, DC

# Table of Contents

# Introduction

The Official Coding Guidelines for ICD-10-CM are dense, confusing and repetitive. In addition, guidelines related to a single body system may be located in multiple sections of the guidelines. For example, guidelines for coding sepsis and severe sepsis are found in Chapter 1 (Certain Infectious and Parasitic Diseases), Chapter 15 (Pregnancy, Childbirth, and the Puerperium), Chapter 16 (Certain Conditions Originating in the Perinatal Period), and Chapter 18 (Symptoms, Signs and Abnormal Clinical and Laboratory Findings, Not Elsewhere Classified). This book combines all the guidelines that are related to one body system or condition in one place.

This book is an update to the 2016 version and includes the new ICD-10-CM guidelines released October 2016.

This book is designed for use as a supplement to coding textbooks for students and as quick reference for coders working in the field. It clarifies the guidelines using charts to provide step by step directions on how to interpret the guidelines, including codes, definitions and sequencing. Coders should confirm the code selected using the Tabular List in the ICD-10-CM code book.

The introduction to each chapter states where the guidelines listed in that chapter are located in the Official Coding Guidelines and a list of the charts included in the chapter.

There are two types of charts in this book. First are charts that designate a condition or reason for admission, principal diagnosis, additional diagnoses, and other guidelines. The coder moves across the rows to find information about sequencing the codes and other guidelines related to that condition or reason for admission. For example, in the chart for Sequencing of Malignancy Codes, the left hand column is entitled "Reason for Admission." The next column is entitled "Principal Diagnosis." The final column is entitled "Additional Diagnoses." Using this chart, you see that when a patient is admitted for treatment of a secondary malignancy, the principal diagnosis is the secondary malignancy, and an additional diagnosis should be listed for the primary neoplasm if it has not been removed or a personal history code if it has been removed.

The other type of chart is designed to clarify coding for complicated conditions not specifically discussed in the guidelines. For example, the chart Coding Sickle-Cell Conditions, includes X marks in columns if the condition is included in the code. Therefore, the code D57.01 includes sickle-cell with crisis and acute chest syndrome.

# General Guidelines

These tables are taken from the Official Coding Guidelines, Section I.A (Conventions for the ICD-10-CM), Section I.B (General Coding Guidelines), Section II (Selection of Principal Diagnosis), Section III (Reporting Additional Diagnoses), and Section IV (Diagnostic Coding and Reporting Guidelines for Outpatient Services). Included in this chapter are these tables:

1) General Diagnosis Guidelines (Apply to Inpatients and Outpatients)
2) Diagnosis Guidelines – Inpatients.
3) Diagnosis Guidelines – Outpatients
4) Symbols, Abbreviations and Words
5) Notes and Sequencing Phrases

## General Diagnosis Guidelines (Apply to Inpatients and Outpatients)

| Conditions | Coding Guidelines |
|---|---|
| **Sequencing Guidelines** | |
| Complications of surgery and/or medical care | List first code for complication. Provider documentation must state relationship between condition and complication.<br>Do **NOT** assume that a condition that occurs after medical care or surgery is a complication unless otherwise instructed by guidelines. Query provider if unclear |
| Admission/encounter for rehabilitation | |
|    Condition still present | List first code for condition requiring rehabilitation |
|    Condition no longer present | List first an aftercare code |
| Condition listed as acute (subacute) and chronic (acute on chronic) | If Alphabetic Index lists codes for both acute (subacute) and chronic AND both are at the same indent level, list both codes.<br>List first code for acute condition. |
| **Other Guidelines** | |
| Conditions related to <u>previous</u> hospital stay or encounter but have no bearing on current stay | Do **NOT** list code for condition<br>List history code if appropriate |
| Borderline condition | Find Alphabetic Index main term Borderline OR<br>Main term for condition and look for subterm Borderline -<br>•   If subterm is listed, list that code.<br>•   If no indented term for condition, list code as if condition confirmed. |
| Signs and symptoms - | |
|    No definitive diagnosis established | List codes for signs and symptoms |
|    Definitive diagnosis established | Signs and symptoms <u>related</u> to definitive diagnosis – do not code<br>Signs and symptoms <u>NOT related</u> to definitive diagnosis – list codes for signs and symptoms in addition to definitive diagnosis |
| Syndromes | Find main term Syndrome in Alphabetic Index.<br>If syndrome is not listed, list codes for manifestations<br>List also codes for manifestations that are not part of syndrome |
| Sequelae | Definition - Late effects or residual effects (condition produced) after acute phase of illness or injury has ended. Example: scar resulting from a burn.<br>No time limit on how long sequelae codes can be used.<br>List first code for current condition, then sequela code unless directed otherwise in Tabular List<br>Do **NOT** list acute code and sequela code for the same condition |
| Laterality | If no code for bilateral - list separate codes for right/left<br>If code for bilateral – use bilateral code<br>•   If each side is treated during separate encounters, code as bilateral for both encounters<br>•   If condition no longer exists on one side during subsequent encounter, code as unilateral |
| Combination codes | Definition - A single code is listed to report:<br>1)  Two diagnoses<br>2)  A diagnosis and associated secondary process (manifestation) or<br>3)  A diagnosis with an associated complication<br>List the combination code only. Do not list each diagnosis separately. |

**CONTINUED ON NEXT PAGE**

# General Diagnosis Guidelines (Apply to Inpatients and Outpatients)

| Conditions | Coding Guidelines |
|---|---|
| Body Mass Index (BMI) (Z68-) | BMI code may be based on documentation from clinicians other than physician, such as a dietician<br>Associated diagnoses such as overweight or obesity must be based on documentation by provider.<br>If conflict between diagnoses, query provider.<br>Code is never listed first |
| Non-pressure ulcers of skin (L98.-) | Code for depth of non-pressure ulcer may be based on documentation from clinicians other than physician, such as a nurse.<br>Associated diagnoses such as presence of ulcer must be based on documentation by provider.<br>If conflict between diagnoses, query provider |
| Pressure ulcers (L89-) | Code for stage of pressure ulcer may be based on documentation from clinicians other than physician, such as a nurse.<br>Presence of ulcer must be based on documentation by provider.<br>If conflict between diagnoses, query provider |
| Coma scale (R40.2-) | Code first condition related to coma – skull fracture, intracranial injury traumatic brain injury, sequelae of cerebrovascular disease or other nontraumatic conditions<br>Code for scale may be based on documentation from clinicians other than physician, such as emergency medical technician<br>Presence of coma must be based on documentation by provider.<br>If conflict between diagnoses, query provider<br>Code is never listed first |
| NIHSS Stroke Scale (R29.7-) | Code first acute stroke (I63)<br>Code for scale may be based on documentation from clinicians other than physician<br>Presence of stroke must be based on documentation by provider.<br>If conflict between diagnoses, query provider<br>Code is never listed first<br>May be recorded more than once during hospitalization |

# Diagnosis Guidelines - Inpatients

| Conditions/Circumstances | Coding Guidelines |
|---|---|
| Patient in acute care, short-term, long term care, hospice, and psychiatric hospital facilities | Patients covered by inpatient guidelines |
| Condition established after study to be chiefly responsible for occasioning admission of patient to the hospital for care | Definition of principal diagnosis |
| Condition requires: <br> 1. Clinical evaluation <br> 2. Therapeutic treatment or diagnostic procedures <br> 3. Extended length of hospital stay <br> 4. Increased nursing care and/or monitoring | Definition of additional diagnosis <br> Do not list codes for conditions related to a previous episode of care which have no bearing on current hospital stay. |
| **Sequencing Guidelines** | |
| Comparative or contrasting conditions (either/or, diagnosis 1 vs. diagnosis 2) | List codes for both conditions as if confirmed. <br> Either diagnosis may be principal diagnosis depending on circumstances unless indicated otherwise in Alphabetic Index or Tabular List |
| Two or more interrelated conditions, each meet definition of principal diagnosis | List codes for both conditions. <br> Either diagnosis may be principal diagnosis |
| Original plan not carried out (patient admitted for surgery but it was not done) | List as principal diagnosis the reason that patient was admitted (reason surgery was going to be done) |
| Patient admitted FROM observation care TO inpatient status | List the condition that led to the admission as principal diagnosis |
| Patient who had outpatient surgery is admitted to post-operative observation unit. Finally admitted TO inpatient status | For admission, list the condition chiefly responsible for admission (usually complication of the surgery) as principal diagnosis |
| Patient admitted FROM outpatient surgery TO inpatient status | Principal diagnosis depends on circumstances of admission: <br> 1. If admitted for complication – principal diagnosis is complication <br> 2. If reason for admission is not documented – principal diagnosis is reason for surgery <br> 3. If reason is unrelated condition – principal diagnosis is unrelated condition |
| **Other Guidelines** | |
| Abnormal findings (laboratory, x-ray, or other diagnostic test results) | Do **NOT** list code unless provider indicates that they are clinically significant. Query provider if necessary. |
| Condition listed on final diagnostic statement (such as discharge summary) AND is related to principal diagnosis | List code for condition |
| Uncertain diagnosis (listed as "probable," "suspected," "likely," "questionable, "possible," or "still to be ruled out") | List code for condition as if confirmed |
| Condition documented as impending or threatened at time of discharge - | |
| Condition did occur | List code for condition |
| Condition did NOT occur | Refer to main terms Impending and/or Threatened in Alphabetic Index-- <br> If condition listed, list that code <br> If condition not listed, code for symptoms |

# Diagnosis Coding - Outpatients

| Condition/Reason for Encounter | Coding Guidelines |
|---|---|
| Patient in outpatient settings such as emergency department, observation unit, outpatient surgery center, and physician offices | Patient covered by outpatient guidelines apply |
| Diagnosis, condition, problem or other reason for encounter/visit shown in the medical record to be chiefly responsible for the services provided | Definition of first-listed diagnosis |
| Coexisting conditions that require or affect patient care, treatment or management | Definition of additional diagnoses |
| **Sequencing Guidelines** | |
| Patient seen for circumstances other than disease or injury (such as routine annual exam) | First-listed diagnosis is Z code (Factors Influencing Health Status and Contact with Health Services) |
| Patient seen for diagnostic services only | First-listed code is condition chiefly responsible for services Additional diagnoses for chronic or other conditions |
| Patient seen for therapeutic services only | First-listed diagnosis is reason therapeutic services were provided Additional diagnoses may be listed as appropriate |
| Patient seen for preoperative evaluation only | First-listed code is from subcategory Z01.81 (encounter for pre-procedural exam) Then list a code for reason procedure will be done Then list a code for any findings from the evaluation |
| Patient seen for ambulatory (outpatient) surgery | First-listed code is reason for surgery. If postoperative diagnosis is different than pre-operative, list post-operative diagnosis only |
| Patient seen for routine exam with abnormal findings | First-listed code is Z00.0- (exam with abnormal findings). Then list a code for the abnormal finding. |
| Outpatient same day surgery | First-listed diagnosis is reason for surgery, even if surgery not carried out |
| Observation stay | First-listed diagnosis is reason for admission to observation |
| Outpatient same day surgery; complication requires admission to observation care | For admission to observation, first-listed diagnosis is reason for surgery. Then list a code for complication |
| **Other Guidelines** | |
| Uncertain diagnosis (listed as "probable," "suspected," "likely," "questionable," "possible," or "still to be ruled out." | Code for signs and symptoms only Do **NOT** code as if confirmed |
| Chronic conditions | May be treated on ongoing basis (multiple visits) List code for each visit as appropriate |
| Laboratory/radiology testing - | |
| Test is routine: patient does not have signs, symptoms or associated diagnosis | Results NOT available – list code Z01.89 (Encounter for other specified special examination) Results ARE available (Provider documented results) – list code for any confirmed or definitive condition. Do **NOT** code signs or symptoms |
| Visit includes 2 tests – a routine test and a nonroutine test (to evaluate sign, symptom or diagnose a condition) | List diagnosis codes for both routine test (Z codes) and reason for nonroutine test (sign, symptom or diagnosis) |

## Symbols, Abbreviations and Words

| Symbol or Words | | Location(s) | Coding Guidelines |
|---|---|---|---|
| ( ) | Parentheses | Alphabetic Index and Tabular List | Encloses supplementary words that may or may not be documented. Whether term is present or not does not affect the code selection. Also called nonessential modifiers |
| [ ] | Brackets | Tabular List Alphabetic Index | In Tabular List - Enclose synonyms, alternative wording or explanatory phrases<br>In Alphabetic Index - Indicates manifestation codes. For example: Code A [Code B]. Both codes must be listed in this order. |
| X | Placeholder | Tabular List | Used with codes that require a 7$^{th}$ character but the code has less than 6 characters.<br>The placeholder X moves the 7$^{th}$ character to the 7$^{th}$ place. |
| NEC | Not elsewhere classified | Alphabetic Index | Means "Other specified" or "Other."<br>Documentation is too detailed. No specific code exists that matches the documentation. |
| NOS | Not otherwise classified | Tabular List | Means "Unspecified."<br>Documentation is not detailed enough to select between several different codes.<br>Do not list a code for a more specific code if it is not supported by the documentation |
| And | | Tabular List | Means either "and" or "or." Documentation may include one or both conditions listed |
| With | | Alphabetic Index | Means "associated with," "due to."<br>Listed as first indented term under main term (not in alphabetical order)<br>A relationship between the conditions is assumed unless documentation states otherwise |
| See | | Alphabetic Index | Main term refers coder to another main term |
| See also | | Alphabetic Index | Main term includes some indented codes but the coder is also referred to another main term |
| Default code | | Alphabetic Index | Code listed next to main term<br>Listed when none of the indented codes matches the documentation |

# Notes and Sequencing Phrases Following Code or Code Category

## in Tabular List

| Inclusion and Exclusion Notes and Terms | |
|---|---|
| Includes notes | Defines or gives examples of what is included in code category. |
| Inclusion Terms | List of conditions coded using that code.<br>List does not include all possible conditions that can be reported using this code |
| Excludes1 notes | Means "not coded here"<br>Code listed in excludes1 note cannot be used with code listed above it.<br>List only one code<br>Exception: If two conditions are unrelated, then list codes for both.<br>If unclear whether conditions are related, query the provider |
| Excludes2 notes | Means "not included here"<br>The condition listed in the note is not part of code listed above it.<br>If both conditions are documented, list 2 codes |
| **Sequencing Phrases - Examples** | |
| Under Code A is note: "Code first B" | List first code B, then code A |
| Under Code C is note: "Use additional code D" | List first code C, then code D |
| Under code E is note: "Use additional code F if applicable" | List first code E, then code F if condition is documented |
| Under code G is note: "Use additional code H to identify causative organism" | List first code G, then Code H if organism that caused the condition (such as bacteria or virus) is known |
| Under code J is note: "Code first underlying disease such as code K" | List first code K, then code J |
| Under code L is note: "Code also code M" | List both codes L and M.<br>Sequencing depends on circumstances |

# Chapter 1

## Certain Infectious and Parasitic Diseases

These tables are taken from the Official Coding Guidelines, Section I.C.1 (Chapter 1: Certain Infectious and Parasitic Diseases); Section I.C.18 (Chapter 18: Symptoms, Signs, and Abnormal Clinical and Laboratory Findings, Not Elsewhere Classified); and Section I.C.21 (Chapter 21: Factors Influencing Health Status and Contact With Health Services).

Included in this chapter are these tables:

1) General Coding Guidelines
2) HIV/AIDS Coding
3) HIV/AIDS Testing
4) Infection Coding for Specific Conditions
5) Coding Sepsis/Severe Sepsis
6) Coding Complications Related to Sepsis/Severe Sepsis
7) Documentation of Sepsis/Severe Sepsis
8) Coding MRSA (Methicillin Resistant Staphylococcus Aureus)
9) Coding MSSA (Methicillin Susceptible Staphylococcus Aureus)

### General Coding Guidelines

| Code Categories | Definition | Coding Guidelines |
|---|---|---|
| Combination codes | Codes that indicate both the infection and the bacteria or virus that caused the infection | List only 1 code.<br>For example: Z37.00 (whooping cough due to Bordetella pertussis without pneumonia) |
| Noncombination codes | Codes that do NOT include both the infection and the bacteria or virus that caused the infection | List first code for the disease<br>Then list code from B95-B97 (bacterial & viral infectious agents as cause of diseases classified elsewhere)<br>For example: chronic obstructive pulmonary disease with streptococcus group B infection. List first J44.0 and then B95.2 |
| Contact/Exposure Z20-, Z77 | Patient has no signs or symptoms of condition but is suspected to have been exposed to it by:<br>1) close personal contact with infected individual or<br>2) having been in an area where disease is epidemic | May be listed first as reason for encounter for testing OR<br>May be listed as additional code to identify potential risk |
| Inoculations and vaccinations Z23 | Prophylactic inoculation | If performed during routine preventive visit (such as well-baby visit), list this code second<br>List also procedure codes for administration of vaccine and types of immunization given |

# HIV/AIDS Coding

| Reason for Admission | Principal Diagnosis | Secondary Diagnoses |
|---|---|---|
| Suspected HIV/AIDS | Code for signs or symptoms. | |
| Confirmed HIV/AIDS | List code B20 or Z21. Condition must be confirmed by physician | |
| Treatment of condition related to HIV/AIDS | Code B20 | Related condition(s) |
| Treatment of condition NOT related to HIV/AIDS | Unrelated condition | Code B20 if patient has symptoms of HIV/AIDS<br>Code Z21 if patient does not now AND has never had symptoms of HIV/AIDS<br>Then code any symptoms if documented |
| Treatment of pregnant patient with HIV/AIDS | Code O98.7- | Code B20 if patient has symptoms of HIV/AIDS<br>Code Z21 if patient does not now AND has never had symptoms of HIV/AIDS<br>Then code any symptoms if documented |
| Treatment of AIDS | Code B20 | Code(s) for manifestations of AIDS |

# HIV/AIDS Testing

| Reason for Admission | Principal Diagnosis | Secondary Diagnoses |
|---|---|---|
| Initial HIV Test | Code Z11.4 | Code Z71.7 (counseling) if done<br>Any signs or symptoms of HIV if present |
| **Patient Seen to Receive Test Results** | | |
| Results are negative | Code Z71.7 (counseling) | Any signs or symptoms of HIV if present |
| Results are positive | Code Z21 or B20 | Any signs or symptoms of HIV if present |
| Results are inconclusive | Code R75 (inclusive lab evidence of HIV) | Any signs or symptoms of HIV if present |

# Infection Coding for Specific Conditions

| Condition | Code | Coding Guidelines |
|---|---|---|
| Zika virus | A92.5 | Code only if documented as confirmed by provider. If not documented, code for symptoms or code for exposure to (Z20.828) |
| H1N1 or H3N2 not identified as novel or variant | J10- | Code only if documented as confirmed by provider. If not documented, list code from J11 |
| Avian influence or other novel influenza A (includes avian, bird and swine flu) | J09- | Code only if documented as confirmed by provider. If not documented, list code from J11 |

For other infections, list code for infection if physician documents condition as "suspected, possible, or probable" for inpatients.

# Coding Sepsis/Severe Sepsis

| Condition/Circumstances | Definition | Guidelines |
|---|---|---|
| **Sepsis/Severe Sepsis due to Infectious Process** | | |
| Sepsis | Sepsis due to systemic infection | List code for underlying infection<br>Then list code for localized infection if present<br>Do **NOT** list code from R65 category |
| Severe sepsis | Sepsis due to systemic infection with acute organ dysfunction | List first code for systemic infection<br>Then list code R65.2-<br>Then list code for associated organ dysfunction and localized infection if present |
| Sepsis with associated organ dysfunction | Code as severe sepsis | List first code for underlying infection<br>Then list code R65.2-<br>Then list code for organ dysfunction |
| Sepsis and organ dysfunction, not documented as related conditions | Organ dysfunction may or may not be due to sepsis | Query provider |
| Patient admitted with sepsis with localized infection | Infection confined to one organ system or area of body | List first code for underlying infection<br>Then list code for localized infection<br>Then list code R65.2- if severe sepsis |
| Patient admitted with localized infection which develops into sepsis after admission | Localized infection spreads to other areas during hospitalization | List first code for localized infection<br>Then list code for systemic infection<br>Then list code R65.2- if severe sepsis |
| Septic Shock | Cardiovascular system failure. Assume this is severe sepsis | List first code for systemic infection<br>Then list code R65.21<br>Then list code for associated organ dysfunction |
| **Sepsis due to Non-Infectious Process** | | |
| Sepsis due to **non-infectious** process (SIRS) | Patient diagnosed with trauma, neoplasm, pancreatitis, burn or other injury. Injury leads to systemic infection | Depends on reason for admission.<br>List first trauma, neoplasm, pancreatitis or injury OR resulting systemic infection as appropriate.<br>Then list code R65.1-<br>Then code organ dysfunction if appropriate. |

List only one code from category R65

R65 code can <u>never</u> be listed as principal diagnosis

# Coding Complications Related to Sepsis/Severe Sepsis

| Reason for admission | Definition | Coding Guidelines |
|---|---|---|
| Bacterial sepsis of newborn | Includes congenital sepsis. | List first code P36-<br>Then list code for systemic infection from B95-B96 IF the P36 code description does not include the bacteria or virus that caused the infection<br>Then list code for severe sepsis if documented (R65.2-)<br>Then list code for any organ dysfunction<br>If newborn's record does not state sepsis as congenital or community-acquired, list code for congenital |
| Postprocedural sepsis/severe sepsis | Systemic infection following a surgical procedure | Sepsis must be documented as due to procedure<br>List first code for complication (such as T8Ø.2-, T81.4-, T88.Ø-, T86. Ø-)<br>Then list code for systemic infection<br>Then list code for severe sepsis and/or septic shock if documented (R65.2)<br>Then list code for any organ dysfunction |
| Pregnancy with septicemia, SIRS, sepsis/severe sepsis, or septic shock | Sepsis in pregnancy | List first code O98.81-<br>Then list code for systemic infection<br>Then list code for severe sepsis if documented (R65.2)<br>Then list code for any organ dysfunction |
| Puerperal sepsis | Sepsis following delivery | List first code O85 Puerperal sepsis<br>Then list code for systemic infection from B95-B96<br>Then list code for severe sepsis if documented (R65.2)<br>Then list code for any organ dysfunction<br>Do **NOT** list codes A40 or (streptococcal sepsis) or A41 (other sepsis) with this code |

# Documentation of Sepsis/Severe Sepsis

| Documentation | Explanation | Coding Guidelines |
|---|---|---|
| Negative or inconclusive blood culture for sepsis | Negative blood culture results do NOT necessarily mean that the patient does not have sepsis | Query physician |
| Urosepsis | A nonspecific term without a diagnosis code. | Query physician |
| Acute organ dysfunction NOT clearly associated with sepsis | Organ dysfunction may be due to a condition other than the sepsis | Query physician |

## Coding MRSA (Methicillin Resistant Staphylococcus Aureus)

| Condition | Principal Diagnosis | Secondary Diagnoses | Do NOT Code |
|---|---|---|---|
| **MRSA Infection** | | | |
| MRSA infection that has combination code | Combination code Example: A41.02 (sepsis due to MRSA) | None | B95.62 (MRSA as cause of disease classified elsewhere) Z16.11 (resistance to penicillins) |
| MRSA infection that does NOT have combination code | Current MRSA infection A49.02 | B95.62 (MRSA as cause of disease classified elsewhere) | Z16.11 (resistance to penicillins) |
| **MRSA Colonization** | | | |
| Colonization - patient NOT currently sick | Z22.322 (carrier or suspected carrier of MRSA) | | Code for infection (patient does not now have infection) |
| Colonization – patient has current MRSA infection | Current MRSA infection | Z22.322 (carrier or suspected carrier of MRSA) | |

## Coding MSSA (Methicillin Susceptible Staphylococcus Aureus)

| Condition | Principal Diagnosis | Secondary Diagnoses | Do NOT Code |
|---|---|---|---|
| **MSSA Infection** | | | |
| MSSA infection that has combination code | Combination code Example: A41.01 (sepsis due to MSSA) | None | B95.61 (MSSA as cause of disease classified elsewhere) Z16.11 (resistance to penicillins) |
| MSSA that does NOT have combination code | Current MSSA infection (A49.01) | B95.61 (MSSA as cause of disease classified elsewhere) | Z16.11 (resistance to penicillins) |
| **MSSA Colonization** | | | |
| Colonization - patient NOT currently sick | Z22.321 (carrier or suspected carrier of MSSA) | | Code for infection (patient does not now have infection) |
| Colonization – patient has current MSSA infection | Current MSSA infection | Z22.321 (carrier or suspected carrier of MSSA) | |

# Chapter 2

## Neoplasms

These tables are taken from the Official Coding Guidelines, Section I.C.2 (Chapter 2: Neoplasms); Section I.C.6 (Chapter 6: Diseases of Nervous System); and Section I.C.21 (Chapter 21: Factors Influencing Health Status and Contact with Health Services).

Included in this chapter are these tables:

1) Definitions of Terms in Neoplasm Table
2) Coding Neoplasms
3) Sequencing Codes for Malignant Neoplasms
4) Subsequent Visits for Neoplasm Treatment
5) Coding Complications Related to Malignant Neoplasms

### Definitions of Terms Used in the Neoplasm Table

| Term | Definition |
|---|---|
| Malignant, primary | Original location where cancer was diagnosed |
| Malignant, secondary | Metastatic cancer |
| Ca in situ | Cancer that has not spread to nearby tissue |
| Benign | Noncancerous growth |
| Uncertain behavior | Tissue has some characteristics of benign cells but also some characteristics of cancerous cells. Documented as uncertain behavior by a pathologist |
| Unspecified behavior | Documentation does not indicate malignant or benign |

### Using the Neoplasm Table

| Type of Neoplasm | Coding Guidelines |
|---|---|
| Neoplasm of a specific organ/tissue | Refer directly to Neoplasm Table |
| Neoplasm described using histological term<br><br>For example: Adenoma, sarcoma, myeloma | Look up histological term in Alphabetic Index.<br>If entry states: "See also Neoplasm by site" and lists a type of neoplasm (benign/malignant/in situ):<br>1) Turn to the Neoplasm Table<br>2) Find the site<br>Then refer to column for type of neoplasm |

# Malignancy Guidelines

| Condition | Coding Guidelines |
|---|---|
| Malignancy of overlapping, contiguous sites | Coding depends on whether or not there is a code for both sites<br>1. One code for both sites. List only 1 code.<br>   For example: carcinoma in situ, rectum and colon – D01.1<br>2. No code for both sites. List malignancy code with 4th digit 8.<br>   For example: Primary malignancy of pleura, overlapping lesion with heart or mediastinum – C38.8 |
| Multiple malignancies, sites are not overlapping or contiguous | List separate codes for each site<br>For example: different quadrants of same breast |
| Malignancy of ectopic tissue | List code for site of origin<br>Example: Ectopic pancreatic malignancy involving stomach. Code to pancreas, not stomach |
| Malignancy previously excised, no further treatment or evidence of condition | List code for history of malignancy (Z85 category)<br>List code for secondary neoplasm if appropriate |
| Secondary malignancy<br>Primary site previously excised with no evidence of condition | List first code for secondary malignancy<br>Then code history code for primary malignancy (Z85 category) |
| Disseminated malignant malignancy, unspecified | List code C80.0 only when patient has advanced metastatic disease AND primary or secondary sites are unknown |
| Primary malignant malignancy, site unspecified | List code C80.1 when primary site cannot be determined<br>Rarely used in inpatient setting |
| Leukemia, multiple myeloma and malignant plasma cell neoplasm | List code from categories C90-C94. Codes indicate whether in remission or not.<br>History of leukemia – Z85.6<br>If unclear whether code for in remission, not in remission or personal history should be used, query provider. |
| Prophylactic organ removal (Z40-) | Normal tissue removed due to genetic susceptibility or family history of malignancy<br>List first code Z40-<br>Then list code for susceptibility or family history if appropriate<br>If patient had malignancy of one site and is having prophylactic removal at another site to prevent new malignancy or metastatic disease, code first Z40.0 and then code for malignancy<br>Do **NOT** list code Z40.0 if patient is having organ removal for treatment of malignancy (not prophylactic) |

# Sequencing Codes for Malignant Neoplasms

| Reason for Admission | Principal Diagnosis | Additional Diagnoses |
|---|---|---|
| Treatment of primary malignancy | Primary malignancy | Secondary neoplasm if documented |
| Treatment of secondary malignancy | Secondary malignancy | Primary neoplasm If not removed Personal history of malignancy if primary malignancy has been removed or treatment completed (Z85-) |
| Recurrence of malignancy | Malignancy code | |
| To determine extent of malignancy (Encounter may include diagnostic procedures) | Malignancy code | Therapy code Z51- if provided during visit |
| Treatment of malignancy in pregnant patient | Code O9A.1- | Malignancy code |
| Chemotherapy, immunotherapy, or radiation therapy No treatment of malignancy | Therapy code Z51- If more than one type of therapy provided, code each | Malignancy code |
| Treatment of malignancy and chemotherapy, immunotherapy or radiation therapy also provided | Malignancy code | Therapy code (Z51-) If more than one type of therapy provided, list code for each type |
| Chemotherapy immunotherapy or radiation therapy Complication develops during encounter | Therapy code Z51- | Complication code Code for neoplasm |

# Subsequent Visits for Neoplasm Treatment

| Reason for Admission | Definition | Coding Guidelines |
|---|---|---|
| Aftercare visit | Treatment of neoplasm has been completed Patient now seen for continued care during healing or recovery process | List code Z51 (aftercare code) May include radiation, immunotherapy or chemotherapy Code also for neoplasm |
| Follow-up visit | Treatment of neoplasm has been completed | List code Z08 (follow-up code) If condition is found to have reoccurred, list code for neoplasm instead of follow-up code |
| Multiple visits for existing neoplasm | Continuing treatment of existing condition | List neoplasm code as many times as necessary Do **NOT** list signs/symptoms instead |

# Coding Complications Related to Malignant Neoplasms

| Reason for Admission | Principal Diagnosis | Additional Diagnoses |
|---|---|---|
| **Anemia due to Malignancy or Treatment** | | |
| Treatment of anemia due to malignancy (Only anemia is treated) | Malignancy code | Anemia in neoplastic disease (D63.0) |
| Treatment of anemia due to chemotherapy (Only anemia is treated) | Anemia due to chemotherapy (D64.81) | Malignancy code Adverse effect of drug (T45.1x5-) |
| Treatment of anemia due to immunotherapy (Only anemia is treated) | Other specified anemia (D64.89) | Malignancy code Adverse effect of drug (T45.1x5-) |
| Treatment of anemia due to radiotherapy (Only anemia is treated) | Other specified anemia (D64.89) | Malignancy code External cause code Y84.2 |
| Treatment of anemia due to malignancy AND treatment of the malignancy | Malignancy code | Anemia in neoplastic disease (D63.0) |
| Treatment of anemia due to both treatment AND the malignancy | Malignancy code | Adverse effect of drug (T45.1x5-) |
| Chemotherapy, immunotherapy or radiotherapy Patient develops anemia during encounter | Therapy code Z51- | Anemia (D64.81) |
| **Dehydration due to Malignancy or Treatment** | | |
| Treatment of dehydration due to malignancy (Only dehydration is treated) | Dehydration (E86.0) | Malignancy code |
| Treatment of dehydration due to chemotherapy (Only dehydration is treated) | Dehydration (E86.0) | Malignancy code Adverse effect of drug (T45.1x5-) |
| Treatment of dehydration due to malignancy AND treatment of the malignancy | Malignancy code | Dehydration (E86.0) |
| Treatment of dehydration due to chemotherapy AND treatment of the malignancy | Malignancy code | Dehydration (E86.0) Adverse effect of drug (T45.1x5-) |
| Chemotherapy, immunotherapy or radiotherapy Patient develops dehydration during encounter | Therapy code Z51- | Dehydration (E86.0) |
| **Fracture due to Malignancy** | | |
| Treatment for fracture due to malignancy (only fracture is treated) | Pathological fracture (M84.5-) | Malignancy code |
| Treatment of malignancy AND fracture | Malignancy code | Pathological fracture (M84.5-) |
| **Pain due to Malignancy** | | |
| Pain related to malignancy (Only pain control or pain management provided) | Malignancy-related pain (G89.3) | Malignancy code |
| Treatment of malignancy and malignancy-related pain | Malignancy code | Malignancy-related pain (G89.3) |
| **Other Complications** | | |
| Malignancy of transplanted organ | Complication code (T86.-) | Malignancy of transplanted organ (C80.2) Malignancy code for specific site |
| Complications of surgical treatment of malignancy | Complication code | Malignancy code or history of malignancy code |
| Pleural effusion due to malignancy | Malignancy | Effusion (J91.0) |
| Malignant ascites | Malignancy | Ascites (R18.0) |
| Chemotherapy, immunotherapy or radiotherapy Patient develops complication during encounter | Therapy code Z51- | Complication code Malignancy code |
| Other complications | Complication code | Malignancy code |

# Chapter 3

# Diseases of the Blood and Blood-forming Organs and Certain Disorders Involving the Immune System

There are no official coding guidelines specifically for this chapter. However, guidelines are included from Section I.C.2.c.1) (Chapter 2: Neoplasms, coding and sequencing of complications, anemia associated with malignancy). Other tables have been included for areas that often cause confusion.

Included in this chapter are these tables:

1) Anemia Related to Malignancy
2) Examples – Conditions that May Be Acquired, Congenital or Perinatal
3) Coding Sickle-cell Conditions

## Anemia Related to Malignancy

| Reason for Admission | Principal Diagnosis | Additional Diagnoses |
|---|---|---|
| Treatment of anemia due to malignancy (Only anemia is treated) | Malignancy code | Anemia in neoplastic disease (D63.0) |
| Treatment of anemia due to chemotherapy (Only anemia is treated) | Anemia due to chemotherapy (D64.81) | Malignancy code Adverse effect of drug (T45.1x5-) |
| Treatment of anemia due to immunotherapy (Only anemia is treated) | Other specified anemia (D64.89) | Malignancy code Adverse effect of drug (T45.1x5-) |
| Treatment of anemia due to radiotherapy (Only anemia is treated) | Other specified anemia (D64.89) | Malignancy code External cause code Y84.2 |
| Treatment of anemia due to treatment AND the malignancy | Malignancy code | Malignancy code Adverse effect of drug (T45.1x5-) |
| Chemotherapy, immunotherapy or radiotherapy Patient develops anemia during encounter | Therapy code Z51- | Anemia (D64.81) |

## Examples – Conditions that May Be Acquired, Congenital, or Perinatal

| Condition | Congenital | Perinatal | Acquired |
|---|---|---|---|
| Aplastic anemia | D61.09 | | D61.3 (idiopathic) |
| Blood loss anemia | | P61.3 | D50.0 |
| Hemolytic anemia | D58.9 | | D59.9 |
| Hemophilia | D66 | | D68.311 |
| Sideroblastic anemia | D64.0 | | D64.1-D64.2 |
| Erythroblastic anemia | D56.1 | P55.9 | |

## Coding Sickle-Cell Conditions

| Code | With crisis | Without crisis | With acute chest syndrome | With splenic sequestration | Unspecified |
|---|---|---|---|---|---|
| Sickle Cell/Hb-55 Disease | | | | | |
| D57.00 | X | | | | X |
| D57.01 | X | | X | | |
| D57.02 | X | | | X | |
| D57.1 | | X | | | |
| Sickle-Cell/Hb-C Disease | | | | | |
| D57.20 | | X | | | |
| D57.211 | X | | X | | |
| D57.212 | X | | | X | |
| D57.219 | X | | | | X |
| D57.3 | | | | | X |
| Sickle Cell Thalassemia | | | | | |
| D57.40 | | X | | | |
| D57.411 | X | | X | | |
| D57.412 | X | | | X | |
| D57.419 | X | | | | X |
| Other Sickle-cell Disorders | | | | | |
| D57.80 | | X | | | |
| D57.811 | X | | X | | |
| D57.812 | X | | | X | |
| D57.819 | X | | | | x |

Crisis – sickle-shaped red blood cells block flow of blood in small blood vessels

Acute chest syndrome – Lung-related complication that can lower levels of oxygen in blood

Splenic sequestration – sickle cell red blood cells become trapped in the spleen, resulting in enlargement and damage to spleen

Sickle cell trait (D57.3) - patient is carrier of sickle cell disease but does not have any symptoms of the condition

# Chapter 4

# Endocrine, Nutritional, and Metabolic Diseases

These tables are taken from the Official Coding Guidelines, Section I.C.4 (Chapter 4: Endocrine, Nutritional and Metabolic Diseases); Section I.C.15 (Chapter 15: Pregnancy, Childbirth and the Puerperium); and Section I.C.19.e (Chapter 19, Adverse Effects, Poisoning, Underdosing and Toxic Effects). Guidelines for documenting Body Mass Index were taken from Section I.B.14 (General Coding Guidelines).

Included in this chapter are these tables:

1) Types of Diabetes Mellitus
2) Coding Guidelines for Diabetes Mellitus
3) Coding Guidelines for Obesity and Overweight

## Types of Diabetes Mellitus

| Code Category | Description | Examples |
|---|---|---|
| **Primary Diabetes** | | |
| E10 | Type 1 | Brittle diabetes<br>Due to autoimmune process<br>Due to immune mediated islet beta cell destruction<br>Idiopathic diabetes<br>Juvenile onset diabetes<br>Ketone-prone diabetes |
| E11 | Type 2 | Diabetes NOS<br>Type of diabetes not documented<br>Diabetes due to insulin secretory diabetes<br>Insulin resistant diabetes |
| **Secondary Diabetes –**<br>**Patient had another condition (first) that caused diabetes (second)** | | |
| E08 | Due to underlying condition | Diabetes due to:<br>Congenital rubella    Malnutrition<br>Cushing's syndrome    Pancreatitis<br>Cystic fibrosis    Other diseases of pancreas<br>Malignancy |
| E09 | Drug or chemical induced | Diabetes due to:<br>Use of steroids, cortisones<br>Some environmental causes |
| E13 | Other specified | Diabetes due to:<br>Genetic defects<br>Postpancreatectomy<br>Postprocedural<br>Secondary diabetes NEC |

# Coding Guidelines for Diabetes Mellitus

| Condition | Principal Diagnosis | Secondary diagnoses |
|---|---|---|
| Multiple conditions related to diabetes | List codes for all related conditions<br>List first code for condition that is focus of this visit | Z79.4 – long-term use of insulin if appropriate<br>Z79.84 – long-term use of oral hypoglycemic drugs<br>**Exception**: Type 1 diabetes assumes insulin dependence. No Z code is used |
| Type of diabetes undocumented | E11 – type 2 diabetes | Z79.4 – long-term use of insulin if appropriate<br>Z79.84 – long-term use of oral hypoglycemic drugs |
| **Diabetes in Pregnancy** | | |
| Pre-existing diabetes | O24.0 through O24.3, O24.8 | Z79.4 – long-term use of insulin if appropriate<br>Z79.84 – long-term use of oral hypoglycemic drugs |
| Gestational diabetes | O24.4- | If treated with both diet and insulin, code only for use of insulin |
| **Secondary Diabetes – Patient has another condition (first) that caused diabetes (second)** | | |
| Due to underlying condition | Underlying condition | E08 – diabetes due to underlying condition |
| Diabetes due to pancreatectomy | E89.1 postprocedural hypoinsulinemia | E13- Secondary diabetes<br>Z90.41- Acquired absence of pancreas<br>Z79.4 – long-term use of insulin if appropriate<br>Z79.84 – long-term use of oral hypoglycemic drugs |
| Diabetes due to adverse effect of drugs | E09 diabetes | Adverse effect T38.0x5-<br>Z79.4 – long-term use of insulin if appropriate |
| Diabetes due to poisoning or overdose | T38.3x1 Poisoning | E09 Drug or chemical induced diabetes<br>Z79.4 – long-term use of insulin if appropriate<br>Z79.84 – long-term use of oral hypoglycemic drugs |
| **Conditions Due to Insulin Pump Failure** | | |
| Underdosing due to insulin pump failure | T85.6- Mechanical complication | T38.3x6- Underdosing of insulin<br>Type of diabetes (E08-E11, E13)<br>Any associated complications<br>Z79.4 – long-term use of insulin if appropriate<br>Z79.84 – long-term use of oral hypoglycemic drugs |
| Overdosing due to insulin pump failure | T85.6- Mechanical complication | T38.3x1—Poisoning by insulin<br>Type of diabetes (E08-E11, E13)<br>Z79.4 – long-term use of insulin if appropriate<br>Z79.84 – long-term use of oral hypoglycemic drugs |

List code Z79.4 only if long-term use of insulin is documented.

Do not list Z79.4 if insulin given temporarily to bring a patient's blood sugar under control during an encounter.

Do not list Z79.4 code with codes in the E10 (type 1) category.

# Obesity and Overweight Coding Guidelines

| Codes | | Coding Guidelines |
|---|---|---|
| Z68 | Body mass index (BMI) | Code may be based on documentation from clinicians other than physician, such as dietician.<br>Associated conditions such as obesity or overweight must be based on documentation by physician<br>Code is never listed first |
| E66 | Overweight and obesity | Code for must be based on documentation from physician<br>List first E66 code<br>Then list code Z68 for BMI |

# Chapter 5

# Mental, Behavioral and Neurodevelopmental Disorders

These tables are taken from the Official Coding Guidelines, Section I.C.5 (Mental, Behavioral and Neurodevelopmental Disorders) and Section I.C.6.b (Diseases of Nervous System, Pain – Category G89).

Included in this chapter are these tables:

1) Coding Conditions Related to Psychoactive Substances
2) Coding Pain Related to Psychological Factors

## Coding Conditions Related to Psychoactive Substances

| Documentation States - | Coding Guidelines |
|---|---|
| Injury or condition occurred while patient was under the influence of a psychoactive substance | Use, abuse or dependence must be documented by provider. <br> If no documentation, do **NOT** list a code from the mental health chapter |
| In remission | Must be specifically documented as in remission by provider <br> List with codes for dependence with 5th digit 1 |
| Both use and abuse | List code for abuse only |
| Both abuse and dependence | List code for dependence only |
| Both use and dependence | List code for dependence only |
| Use, abuse and dependence | List code for dependence only |

## Coding Pain Related to Psychological Factors

| Condition | Principal Diagnosis | Secondary Diagnoses |
|---|---|---|
| Pain disorders <u>exclusively</u> related to psychological factors | F45.41 | None. Do **NOT** list code from G89 |
| Pain disorders <u>partly</u> related to psychological factors | F45.42 | List code from G89 |
| Mental disorder due to known physiological (physical) factors <br> For example: dementia due to vascular conditions | Underlying condition | Mental condition |

# Chapter 6

## Diseases of the Nervous System

These tables are taken from the Official Coding Guidelines, Section I.C.2 (Neoplasms); Section I.C.5 (Mental, Behavioral and Neurodevelopmental Disorders), Section I.C.6 (Disease of Nervous System); and Section I.C.19 (Injury, Poisoning, and Certain Other Consequences of External Causes). In addition, a table defining terms related to epilepsy is included.

Included in this chapter are these tables:

1) Coding for Seizure and Epilepsy
2) Sequencing Pain Codes
3) Coding for Pain Related to Specific Conditions
4) Coding for Conditions Affecting Dominant/Nondominant Sides
5) Coding for Pain Related to Specific Conditions

# Coding for Seizures and Epilepsy

| Code | Term | Definition and Coding Guidelines |
|---|---|---|
| R56.9 | Seizure or convulsions | Transient disturbance of cerebral function caused by an abnormal paroxysmal (sudden) neuronal discharge in brain. Do **NOT** assume that seizures indicate epilepsy |
| R56.9 | Convulsions | Paroxysmal (sudden), involuntary muscular contractions and relaxations Do **NOT** assume that seizures indicate epilepsy |
| G40- | Epilepsy and recurrent seizures | Disorder with recurrent seizures Must be documented as epilepsy or epileptic syndrome |
| G40.0- G40.2 | Localization-related idiopathic Seizures of localized onset Epilepsy and epileptic syndromes | Seizures involve one area of brain Cause is unknown |
| G40.1- | Simple partial seizure Symptomatic epilepsy and epileptic syndromes | Affects small region of brain No loss of consciousness |
| G40.2- | Complex partial or psychomotor seizure Symptomatic epilepsy and epileptic syndromes | Affects both sides of cerebrum Change in or loss of consciousness |
| G40.3- | Generalized idiopathic Epilepsy and epileptic syndromes | Seizures involve the whole brain at the same time Cause is unknown |
| G40.3- | Tonic-clonic or grand mal | Affects the entire brain Sudden loss of consciousness and falling to the floor. |
| G40.A- | Absence epileptic syndrome | Muscle twitching or jerking for several seconds |
| G40.B- | Juvenile myotonic epilepsy | Jerking and twitching in upper body, arms or legs |
| G40.4- | Other generalized epilepsy and epileptic syndromes | Included grand mal seizures NOS Nonspecific epileptic seizures |
| G40.5- | Epileptic seizures due to external causes | Cause may be alcohol, drugs, or stress List also epilepsy and seizures (G40-) Sequencing of code G40.5 depends on circumstances of visit List additional code for adverse effect to identify drug if appropriate (T36-T50 with 5th or 6th digit 5) |
| G40.8- | Other epilepsy and recurrent seizures | Includes epilepsy and epileptic syndromes undetermined as to whether focal or generalized |
| G40.9- | Epilepsy, unspecified | Not enough documentation to select a more specific code |
| 5th digit | Intractable | Difficult to manage or control (treatment not working) May be documented as: 1) Pharmacoresistant (resistant to treatment with drugs) 2) Treatment resistant 3) Refractory (medically) or 4) Poorly controlled |
| 6th digit | Status epilepticus | Prolonged seizure (more than 30 minutes) or a series of repeated seizures without regaining consciousness |
| Z82.0 | Family history of epilepsy | Member of patient's family has or had epilepsy. Code used to justify extra tests or visits |

## Sequencing Pain Codes

| Reason for Admission | Principal Diagnosis | Secondary Diagnoses |
|---|---|---|
| Pain control/pain management | Pain – G89 | List code for specific site if known<br>List code for underlying cause if known |
| Insertion of neurostimulator to treat pain<br>No treatment for underlying condition | Pain – G89 | List code for underlying condition |
| Pain, definitive diagnosis known | Definitive diagnosis | List code for pain if code provides additional information (such as acute or chronic) |
| Procedure to treat underlying condition AND neurostimulator inserted to treat pain<br>Cause of pain is known | Underlying condition | List code for pain – G89 |
| Any reason other than pain control<br>No definitive cause of pain established | Site of pain | List code for pain – G89 |
| Treatment of underlying condition | Underlying condition | Do **NOT** list code for pain – G89 |
| Treatment of pain disorder with related psychological factors | List code F45.42 and a code from category G89<br>Sequencing depends on circumstances of visit | |

If pain is not documented as acute, chronic, post-thoracotomy, postprocedural or neoplasm-related, do not list a G89 code.

There is no set timeframe for when pain is considered acute and when it is considered chronic. Use documentation of acute or chronic from provider.

## Coding for Pain Related to Specific Conditions

| Reason for Admission | Principal Diagnosis | Secondary Diagnoses |
|---|---|---|
| **Pain Related to Neoplasms** | | |
| Pain control management<br>No treatment of neoplasm | Pain – G89.3 | Neoplasm |
| Treatment of neoplasm AND pain | Neoplasm | Pain – G89.3 |
| **Postoperative Pain** | | |
| Pain NOT associated with post-op complication | Pain – G89.3 | |
| Pain associated with specific post-op complication | Complication code from chapter 19 | Acute pain – G89.1-<br>Chronic pain – G89.2- |
| Pain due to device, implant or graft | Complication code T85.84x- | Site of pain<br>Pain – G89.18 or G89.28 |
| **Other Conditions** | | |
| Central pain syndrome* | G89.0 | |
| Chronic pain syndrome** | G89.4 | |

*Central pain syndrome is damage or dysfunction of central nervous system, often due to stroke, epilepsy or other conditions.

**Chronic pain syndrome - pain lasting 3 months or more, affecting multiple body systems and usually unresponsive to treatment. Chronic pain syndrome is not the same as chronic pain.

# Coding for Conditions Affecting Dominant/Nondominant Sides

| Affected Side | Code as - |
|---|---|
| **Patient's *Right* Side Affected** | |
| Patient is right handed | Dominant |
| Patient is left handed | Nondominant |
| No documentation as to whether patient is right or left handed | Dominant |
| Patient is ambidextrous | Dominant |
| **Patient's *Left* Side Affected** | |
| Patient is right handed | Nondominant |
| Patient is left handed | Dominant |
| No documentation as to whether patient is right or left handed | Nondominant |
| Patient is ambidextrous | Dominant |

# Chapter 7

# Diseases of the Eye and Adnexa

These tables are taken from the Official Coding Guidelines, Section I.C.7 (Diseases of Eye and Adnexa). Other tables have been included for areas that often cause confusion.

Included in this chapter are these tables:

1) Coding Guidelines for Glaucoma
2) Coding Bilateral Glaucoma
3) Coding Vision Conditions: Both Eyes Have Same Degree of Impairment
4) Coding Vision Conditions: Eyes Have Different Degrees of Impairment

## Coding Guidelines for Glaucoma*

| Circumstances | Coding Guideline | Comments |
|---|---|---|
| Patient admitted with glaucoma – stage changes during admission | Code highest stage documented | |
| Stage documented as indeterminate | Use 7th character 4 | Physician documents that the stage cannot be clinically determined |
| Unspecified stage | Use 7th character 0 | Documentation does not specify stage |

*List as many codes as needed to fully describe type and stage of glaucoma and affected eye(s)

## Coding Bilateral Glaucoma

| Type of Glaucoma | Coding Guideline | Examples |
|---|---|---|
| **Same Type/Same Stage** | | |
| Unspecified and primary open-angle glaucoma | List one code No digits for right, left or bilateral | H40.11x1 Primary open-angle glaucoma, mild stage |
| Other types of glaucoma | List two codes with digit for right, left, bilateral OR List one code for unspecified | H40.1211 Right eye, low-tension glaucoma, mild H40.1221 Left eye, low-tension glaucoma, mild |
| **Different Types/Different Stages** | | |
| All types of glaucoma | Code each side separately Do **NOT** use bilateral codes | H40.1313 Right eye, pigmentary glaucoma, severe H40.1422 Left eye, capsular glaucoma, moderate |

# Coding Vision Conditions

## Both Eyes Have Same Degree of Impairment

| Condition in Both Eyes | Code |
|---|---|
| Blind | H54.0 |
| Low vision | H54.2 |
| Unqualified (unspecified) | H54.3 |
| Legal blindness | H54.8 |

# Coding Vision Conditions

## Eyes Have Different Degrees of Impairment

| Code | Right Eye | Left Eye |
|---|---|---|
| **Blind/Low vision** | | |
| H54.11 | Blind | Low vision |
| H54.12 | Low vision | Blind |
| H54.10 | Unspecified as to right or left eye | |
| **Blind/Normal Vision** | | |
| H54.41 | Blind | Normal vision |
| H54.42 | Normal vision | Blind |
| H54.40 | Unspecified as to right or left eye | |
| **Low Vision/Normal Vision** | | |
| H54.51 | Low vision | Normal vision |
| H54.52 | Normal vision | Low vision |
| H54.50 | Unspecified as to right or left eye | |
| **Unqualified (Unspecified) Visual Loss** | | |
| H54.61 | Unqualified visual loss | Normal vision |
| H54.62 | Normal vision | Unqualified visual loss |
| H54.60 | Unspecified as to right or left eye | |

# Chapter 8

## Diseases of the Ear and Mastoid Process

There are no official guidelines specifically for this chapter. However, tables have been included for areas that often cause confusion.

Included in this chapter are these tables:

1) Coding Nonsuppurative, Acute/Subacute Serous Otitis Media
2) Coding Nonsuppurative, Chronic Serous Otitis Media
3) Coding Suppurative, Acute Otitis Media
4) Coding Suppurative, Chronic Otitis Media
5) Coding Otitis Media Not Specified as Chronic or Acute
6) Coding Hearing Loss

### Coding *Nonsuppurative, Acute/Subacute* Serous Otitis Media

| Code | Laterality | | | | Type of Otitis Media | | | |
|---|---|---|---|---|---|---|---|---|
| | Right | Left | Bilateral | Unspecified | Recurrent | Mucoid (allergic) | Serous | Other |
| H65.00 | | | | X | | | X | |
| H65.01 | X | | | | | | X | |
| H65.02 | | X | | | | | X | |
| H65.03 | | | X | | | | X | |
| H65.04 | X | | | | X | | X | |
| H65.05 | | X | | | X | | X | |
| H65.06 | | | X | | X | | X | |
| H65.07 | | | | X | X | | X | |
| H65.111 | X | | | | | X | X | |
| H65.112 | | X | | | | X | X | |
| H65.113 | | | X | | | X | X | |
| H65.114 | X | | | | X | X | X | |
| H65.115 | | X | | | X | X | X | |
| H65.116 | | | X | | X | X | X | |
| H65.117 | | | | X | X | X | X | |
| H65.119 | | | | X | | X | X | |
| H65.191 | X | | | | | | | X |
| H65.192 | | X | | | | | | X |
| H65.193 | | | X | | | | | X |
| H65.194 | X | | | | X | | | X |
| H65.195 | | X | | | X | | | X |
| H65.196 | | | X | | X | | | X |
| H65.197 | | | | X | X | | | X |
| H65.199 | | | | X | | | | X |

Codes in subcategory H65.11 have mucoid and serous as nonessential modifiers.

## Coding *Nonsuppurative, Chronic* Otitis Media

| Code | Laterality | | | | Type of Otitis Media | | | | |
|---|---|---|---|---|---|---|---|---|---|
| | Right | Left | Bilateral | Unspecified | Serous | Mucoid | Allergic | Other | Unspecified |
| H65.20 | | | | X | X | | | | |
| H65.21 | X | | | | X | | | | |
| H65.22 | | X | | | X | | | | |
| H65.23 | | | X | | X | | | | |
| H65.30 | | | | X | | X | | | |
| H65.31 | X | | | | | X | | | |
| H65.32 | | X | | | | X | | | |
| H65.33 | | | X | | | X | | | |
| H65.411 | X | | | | | | X | | |
| H65.412 | | X | | | | | X | | |
| H65.413 | | | X | | | | X | | |
| H65.419 | | | | X | | | X | | |
| H65.491 | X | | | | | | | X | |
| H65.492 | | X | | | | | | X | |
| H65.493 | | | X | | | | | X | |
| H65.499 | | | | X | | | | X | |

## Coding *Suppurative, Acute* Otitis Media

| Code | Laterality | | | | Type of Otitis Media | |
|---|---|---|---|---|---|---|
| | Right | Left | Bilateral | Unspecified | Spontaneous Rupture of Ear Drum | Recurrent |
| H66.001 | X | | | | | |
| H66.002 | | X | | | | |
| H66.003 | | | X | | | |
| H66.004 | X | | | | | X |
| H66.005 | | X | | | | X |
| H66.006 | | | X | | | X |
| H66.007 | | | | X | | X |
| H66.009 | | | | X | | |
| H66.011 | X | | | | X | |
| H66.012 | | X | | | X | |
| H66.013 | | | X | | X | |
| H66.014 | X | | | | X | X |
| H66.015 | | X | | | X | X |
| H66.016 | | | X | | X | X |
| H66.017 | | | | X | X | X |
| H66.019 | | | | X | X | |

## Coding *Suppurative, Chronic* Otitis Media

| Code | Laterality | | | | Type of Otitis Media | | |
|------|-------|------|-----------|-------------|----------------|---------------|-------|
|      | Right | Left | Bilateral | Unspecified | Tubotympanic* | Atticoantral** | Other |
| H66.10 |   |   |   | X |   |   |   |
|        |   |   |   |   | X |   |   |
| H66.11 | X |   |   |   | X |   |   |
| H66.12 |   | X |   |   | X |   |   |
| H66.13 |   |   | X |   | X |   |   |
| H66.20 |   |   |   | X |   | X |   |
| H66.21 | X |   |   |   |   | X |   |
| H66.22 |   | X |   |   |   | X |   |
| H66.23 |   |   | X |   |   | X |   |
| H66.3x1 | X |   |   |   |   |   | X |
| H66.3x2 |   | X |   |   |   |   | X |
| H66.3x3 |   |   | X |   |   |   | X |
| H66.3x9 |   |   |   | X |   |   | X |

*Tubotympanic – involves the ear drum and Eustachian tube
**Atticoantral – involves middle ear and mastoid cavity

## Coding Otitis Media – Not Specified as *Acute* or *Chronic*

| Code | Laterality | | | | Type of Otitis Media | | | |
|------|-------|------|-----------|-------------|-----------------|-------------|--------------------------------------|-------|
|      | Right | Left | Bilateral | Unspecified | Non-suppurative | Suppurative | In Diseases Classified Elsewhere* | Other |
| H65.90 |   |   |   | X | X |   |   |   |
| H65.91 | X |   |   |   | X |   |   |   |
| H65.92 |   | X |   |   | X |   |   |   |
| H65.93 |   |   | X |   | X |   |   |   |
| H66.40 |   |   |   | X |   | X |   |   |
| H66.41 | X |   |   |   |   | X |   |   |
| H66.42 |   | X |   |   |   | X |   |   |
| H66.43 |   |   | X |   |   | X |   |   |
| H66.90 |   |   |   | X |   |   |   | X |
| H66.91 | X |   |   |   |   |   |   | X |
| H66.92 |   | X |   |   |   |   |   | X |
| H66.93 |   |   | X |   |   |   |   | X |
| H67.1 | X |   |   |   |   |   | X |   |
| H67.2 |   | X |   |   |   |   | X |   |
| H67.3 |   |   | X |   |   |   | X |   |
| H67.9 |   |   |   | X |   |   | X |   |

*For otitis media in diseases classified elsewhere (category H67), code first underlying disease, such as infection
Code also perforated ear drum if documented (H72 category)

# Coding Hearing Loss

| Code | Right Ear | Left Ear |
|---|---|---|
| **Conductive Hearing Loss** | | |
| H90.1 | Hearing loss | Normal hearing |
| H90.12 | Normal hearing | Hearing loss |
| H90.0 | Bilateral hearing loss | |
| H90.2 | Unspecified as to whether right or left ear affected | |
| **Sensorineural Hearing Loss** | | |
| H90.41 | Hearing loss | Normal hearing |
| H90.42 | Normal hearing | Hearing loss |
| H90.3 | Bilateral hearing loss | |
| H90.5 | Unspecified as to whether right or left ear affected | |
| **Mixed Conductive and Sensorineural Hearing Loss** | | |
| H90.71 | Hearing loss | Normal hearing |
| H90.72 | Normal hearing | Hearing loss |
| H90.6 | Bilateral hearing loss | |
| H90.8 | Unspecified as to whether right or left ear affected | |
| **Ototoxic Hearing Loss*** | | |
| H91.01 | Hearing loss | Normal hearing |
| H91.02 | Normal hearing | Hearing loss |
| H91.03 | Bilateral hearing loss | |
| H91.09 | Unspecified as to whether right or left ear affected | |
| **Presbycusis** | | |
| H91.11 | Hearing loss | Normal hearing |
| H91.12 | Normal hearing | Hearing loss |
| H91.13 | Bilateral hearing loss | |
| H91.10 | Unspecified as to whether right or left ear affected | |
| **Sudden Idiopathic Hearing Loss** | | |
| H91.21 | Hearing loss | Normal hearing |
| H91.22 | Normal hearing | Hearing loss |
| H91.23 | Bilateral hearing loss | |
| H91.20 | Unspecified as to whether right or left ear affected | |
| **Other Specified Hearing Loss** | | |
| H91.8x1 | Hearing loss | Normal hearing |
| H91.8x2 | Normal hearing | Hearing loss |
| H91.8x3 | Bilateral hearing loss | |
| H91.8x9 | Unspecified as to right or left ear affected | |
| **Unspecified Hearing Loss** | | |
| H91.91 | Hearing loss | Normal hearing |
| H91.92 | Normal hearing | Hearing loss |
| H91.93 | Bilateral hearing loss | |
| H91.90 | Unspecified as to right or left ear affected | |

*Ototoxic hearing loss may be due to poisoning or adverse effect.
If due to poisoning, list first a code from T36-T65 with 5th or 6th digit 1-4 or 6 and then ototoxic code.
If due to adverse effect, list ototoxic code first and then code from T36-T50 with fifth or sixth character 5

# Chapter 9

# Diseases of Circulatory System

These tables are taken from the Official Coding Guidelines, Section I.C.9 (Diseases of the Circulatory System) and Section I.C.21 (Factors Influencing Health Status and Contact with Health Services).

Included in this chapter are these tables:

1) Coding for Hypertension
2) Coding for Myocardial Infarction
3) Coding for Heart Conditions
4) Coding for Cerebrovascular Conditions
5) Coding for Hemiplegia, Hemiparesis and Monoplegia Following Cerebrovascular Conditions

# Coding for Hypertension

| Reason for Admission | Coding Guidelines/ Definitions | Principal Diagnosis | Secondary Diagnoses |
|---|---|---|---|
| Uncontrolled hypertension | Untreated hypertension or hypertension not responding to treatment | List code from categories I10-I15 as appropriate | |
| Hypertensive crisis – includes Hypertensive urgency Hypertensive emergency Unspecified hypertensive crisis | Severe increase in blood pressure that can lead to a stroke | List code from category I16 and categories I10-I15 Circumstances of admission determine which code is listed first | |
| Controlled hypertension | Patient with hypertension that is controlled by therapy. | List code from categories I10-I15 as appropriate | |
| Transient hypertension | Do not code as hypertension | List symptom code R03.0 If patient is pregnant, list code from categories O13 or O14 | |
| Secondary hypertension | Code separately for underlying condition and secondary hypertension (I15) | Circumstances of admission determine which code is listed first | |
| Hypertension due to heart disease | Do **NOT** assume conditions are related. Relationship must be documented by physician (using terms such as "due to" or "hypertensive") | Category I11 | Category I50 (heart failure) if documented |
| Hypertension NOT due to heart disease | Code hypertension (I10) and heart disease (I50, I51.4-I51.9) separately | Circumstances of admission determine which code is listed first | |
| Hypertensive cerebrovascular disease | Code each condition separately | Categories I60-I69 | Categories I10-I15 |
| Hypertension and chronic kidney disease | Assume conditions are related unless specifically documented as unrelated. The two conditions are linked by use of the word "with" in the Alphabetic Index | Category I12 | Category N18 Category N17 (renal failure) if documented |
| Hypertension, heart disease and chronic kidney disease | Assume that conditions are related | Category I13 | Category N18 Category I50 (heart failure) if documented |
| Hypertension in pregnancy | Code for pregnancy. See notes under pregnancy codes. | Categories O10-O11, O13-O16 | Code hypertension if there is a "use additional code" note under pregnancy code |
| Intraoperative and post-operative hypertension | Relationship between surgery and hypertension must be documented by physician | Category I97 | Code for specific condition if provides additional information |
| Hypertensive retinopathy | Code retinopathy (H35.0) and hypertension (I10-I15) separately | Circumstances of admission determine which code is listed first | |

# Coding for Myocardial Infarctions

## STEMI and NSTEMI

| Condition | Diagnosis Code |
|---|---|
| AMI not specified as STEMI or NSTEMI or site not specified | Code I21.3 |
| NSTEMI evolves into a STEMI | Code for STEMI (I21.0-I21.3) |
| STEMI converts to NSTEMI due to therapy | Code for STEMI (I21.0-I21.3) |
| Transmural, site not specified | Code I21.3 |
| Non-transmural, with or without specified site | Code I21.4 |
| Subendocardial, with or without specified site | Code I21.4 |

AMI - acute myocardial infarction. May be described as STEMI or NSTEMI.
STEMI - St elevation myocardial infarction. Coronary artery completely blocked by blood clot.
NSTEMI - Non-ST elevation myocardial infarction. Coronary artery partially blocked by blood clot.
Transmural AMI – involves entire thickness of left ventricular wall
Subendocardial AMI – involves only inner 1/3 to ½ of left ventricular wall

# Coding for Heart Conditions

| Reason for Admission | Principal Diagnosis | Secondary Diagnosis |
|---|---|---|
| **Initial Infarction Occurred 4 Weeks Ago or Less (0 to 28 Days)** | | |
| Continued care required | Category I21 | |
| Treatment of subsequent AMI within this time period | Category I22 and category I21<br>Circumstances of admission determine which code is listed first | |
| Treatment of complication of AMI <u>Same admission</u> as initial AMI treatment | Category I21 – initial AMI *OR* Category I22 – subsequent AMI | I23 - complication |
| Treatment of complication of AMI <u>Different admission</u> than initial AMI treatment | Category I23 - complication | Category I21 – initial AMI *OR* Category I22 – subsequent AMI |
| **Infarction Occurred More than 4 Weeks Ago (29 days or more)** | | |
| Continued care required | Z48.812 – aftercare | |
| Continued care NOT required No current symptoms | I25.2 - old myocardial infarction | |
| **Other Guidelines** | | |
| Coronary artery disease with AMI | AMI – I21-I23 as appropriate | Coronary artery disease |
| Atherosclerotic coronary artery disease and angina | Code from category I25 Assume angina and coronary artery disease are related unless documented otherwise. | Do **NOT** code angina (I20) separately |

# Coding for Cerebrovascular Conditions (CVA)

| Condition | Coding Guidelines | Principal Diagnosis | Secondary Diagnosis |
|---|---|---|---|
| Acute stroke (I63) | Use NIHSS codes (R29.7-) with codes from category I63 to identify the patient's neurological status and severity of stroke | I63- | R29.7-<br>May be recorded more than once during hospitalization |
| Sequelae of CVA | Sequelae may be present immediately or at any time after initial CVA | Circumstances of admission determine if this code (I69) is listed first | |
| Sequelae and current cerebrovascular disease | Code for both sequela (Category I69) and current cerebrovascular disease<br>Do **NOT** code I69 if there are no neurologic deficits | Circumstances of admission determine which code is listed first | |
| History of transient ischemic attack and cerebral infarction | Do **NOT** list history code Z86.73 if sequelae (neurologic deficits) are documented | Circumstances of admission determine if this code is listed first | |
| Status post tPA* administration | Used only when patient is in one facility, receives tPA and is then moved to a different facility | Cerebrovascular condition | Z92.82 |
| Hypertensive cerebrovascular disease | Code each condition separately | Categories I60-I69 | Categories I10-I15 |
| Intraoperative or post-procedural infarction or hemorrhage | Relationship between intraoperative or postprocedural condition and CVA must be specifically documented | Code category I97 | Some codes in I97 category include "use additional code" note |

*tPA – tissue plasminogen activator dissolves clots and improves blood flow to brain in cases of stroke. Must be administered within 3-4 hours of onset of CVA.

# Coding for Hemiplegia, Hemiparesis and Monoplegia Following Cerebrovascular Conditions

| Affected Side | Code as - |
|---|---|
| **Patient's *Right* Side Affected** | |
| Patient is right handed | Dominant |
| Patient is left handed | Nondominant |
| No documentation as to whether patient is right or left handed | Dominant |
| Patient is ambidextrous | Dominant |
| **Patient's *Left* Side Affected** | |
| Patient is right handed | Nondominant |
| Patient is left handed | Dominant |
| No documentation as to whether patient is right or left handed | Nondominant |
| Patient is ambidextrous | Dominant |

# Chapter 10

# Diseases of the Respiratory System

These tables are taken from the Official Coding Guidelines, Section I.C.10 (Diseases of the Respiratory System) and Section I.C.21 (Factors Influencing Health Status and Contact with Health Services).

Included in this chapter are these tables:

1) Coding Chronic Obstructive Pulmonary Disease (COPD) and Related Conditions
2) Coding for Respiratory Failure
3) Coding for Certain Influenza Viruses
4) Ventilator-Associated Conditions.

## Coding Chronic Obstructive Pulmonary Disease (COPD)

## and Related Conditions

| Condition | Principal Diagnosis | Secondary Diagnoses |
|---|---|---|
| **COPD** | | |
| COPD, unspecified | J44.9 | |
| COPD with acute lower respiratory infection | J44.0 | Infection |
| COPD with (acute) exacerbation Decompensated COPD* | J44.1 | Infection if documented |
| **Asthma** | | |
| With COPD | J44.9 | Type of asthma (J45-) Infection if applicable |
| Chronic obstructive asthma | J44.9 | Type of asthma (J45-) Infection if applicable |
| Asthma without COPD | J45.2 -J45.5- | |
| **Bronchial Conditions** | | |
| Chronic bronchitis with airways obstruction (Chronic obstructive bronchitis) | J44.9 | Infection if applicable |
| Emphysema with chronic bronchitis (chronic emphysematous bronchitis) | J44- | Infection if applicable |
| Emphysema without chronic bronchitis | J43- | |
| Chronic obstructive tracheobronchitis | J44- | Infection if applicable |
| Simple, mucopurulent chronic bronchitis | J41- | |
| Chronic tracheitis/bronchotracheitis | J42 | |
| Chronic bronchitis NOS | J42 | |
| Bronchiectasis | J47- | |
| **Asthma and Bronchitis** | | |
| Chronic asthmatic (obstructive) bronchitis | J44 | Type of asthma (J45-) Infection if applicable |

**Note**: Most of these code categories have extensive "use additional code" notes

*Acute exacerbation and decompensated COPD – worsening or decompensation of a chronic condition. Not the same as an infection superimposed on a chronic condition, though an exacerbation may be triggered by an infection.

# Coding for Respiratory Failure

| Condition | Principal Diagnosis | Secondary Diagnoses |
|---|---|---|
| Acute respiratory failure (J96.0-) or Respiratory failure acute and chronic (J96.2-) present on admission | List respiratory failure as principal diagnosis if:<br>1. Condition meets definition of principal diagnosis* AND<br>2. Guidelines support this sequencing | |
| Respiratory failure and another acute condition (may or may not be respiratory condition) present on admission | Code for reason for admission. Either may be principal diagnosis if:<br>1. Both conditions equally responsible for admission AND<br>2. Guidelines do not have any sequencing rules<br>If unclear, query provider | |
| Respiratory failure occurs after admission | Reason for admission | Respiratory failure |
| Respiratory failure in pregnant patient | Code from pregnancy chapter | J96 code |
| Respiratory failure in poisoning patient | Code from injury chapter | J96 code |
| Respiratory failure in newborn | Code from newborn chapter | J96 code |

*The principal diagnosis is defined as: "that condition established after study to be chiefly responsible for occasioning the admission of the patient to the hospital for care."

# Coding for Certain Influenza Viruses

| Condition | Code | Coding Guidelines |
|---|---|---|
| H1N1 or H3N2 not identified as novel or variant | J10- | Code only if documented as confirmed by provider. If not documented, list code from J11 |
| Avian influenza or other novel influenza A | J09- | Code only if documented as confirmed by provider. If not documented, list code from J11 |

For other infections, list code for infection if physician documents condition as "suspected, possible, or probable."

# Ventilator Associated Conditions

| Condition | Coding Guideline |
|---|---|
| Ventilator associated pneumonia (VAP) present on admission | List first code J95.851 (VAP)<br>Then list code for organism<br>Do NOT code from J12-J18 for type of pneumonia |
| Patient admitted with one type of pneumonia, develops ventilator-associated pneumonia after admission | List first code for type of pneumonia at admission<br>Then list code J95.851 (VAP) |
| Patient seen for weaning from mechanical ventilator | List first code J96.1- (chronic respiratory failure)<br>Then list code Z99.11 (dependence on respiratory [ventilator] status) |
| Documented pneumonia, patient on ventilator | If documentation does not specifically state pneumonia is associated with ventilator, do NOT code ventilator associated pneumonia (J95.851)<br>If unclear, query provider |
| Postprocedural pneumonia, patient on ventilator | Documentation must specifically state pneumonia is associated with ventilator. If documented list code J95.851 |

# Chapter 11

## Diseases of Digestive System

There are no Official Coding Guidelines specifically for this chapter. Tables have been included for areas that often cause confusion.

Included in this chapter are these tables:

1) Coding for Ulcers
2) Coding for Hernias with Laterality
3) Coding for Other Hernias
4) Coding for Cholecystitis (Inflammation of the Gallbladder)
5) Coding for Cholangitis (Inflammation of the Biliary Tract)
6) Coding for Calculi Only – No Cholecystitis or Cholangitis

# Coding for Ulcers

| Code | Acute | Chronic | Unspecified | Hemorrhage (Bleeding) | Perforation |
|------|-------|---------|-------------|-----------------------|-------------|
| **Gastric (Stomach) Ulcers** | | | | | |
| K25.0 | X | | | X | |
| K25.1 | X | | | | X |
| K25.2 | X | | | X | X |
| K25.3 | X | | | | |
| K25.4 | | X | X | X | |
| K25.5 | | X | X | | X |
| K25.6 | | X | X | X | X |
| K25.7 | | X | | | |
| K25.9 | | | X | | |
| **Duodenal (small intestine) Ulcers** | | | | | |
| K26.0 | X | | | X | |
| K26.1 | X | | | | X |
| K26.2 | X | | | X | X |
| K26.3 | X | | | | |
| K26.4 | | X | X | X | |
| K26.5 | | X | X | | X |
| K26.6 | | X | X | X | X |
| K26.7 | | X | | | |
| K26.9 | | | X | | |
| **Peptic Ulcer (Unspecified Site)** | | | | | |
| K27.0 | X | | | X | |
| K27.1 | X | | | | X |
| K27.2 | X | | | X | X |
| K27.3 | X | | | | |
| K27.4 | | X | X | X | |
| K27.5 | | X | X | | X |
| K27.6 | | X | X | X | X |
| K27.7 | | X | | | |
| K27.9 | | | X | | |
| **Gastrojejunal (stomach and jejunum) Ulcers** | | | | | |
| K28.0 | X | | | X | |
| K28.1 | X | | | | X |
| K28.2 | X | | | X | X |
| K28.3 | X | | | | |
| K28.4 | | X | X | X | |
| K28.5 | | X | X | | X |
| K28.6 | | X | X | X | X |
| K28.7 | | X | | | |
| K28.9 | | | X | | |

If documentation lists peptic ulcer of a specific site, list a code for the site, not a code for peptic ulcer.

Unspecified with hemorrhage (bleeding) – 4th digit 4

Unspecified with perforation – 4th digit 5

Unspecified with hemorrhage (bleeding) and perforation – 4th digit 6

Unspecified without hemorrhage (bleeding) or perforation – 4th digit 9

# Coding for Hernias with Laterality

| Code | Laterality | | Timing | | With Gangrene* | With Obstruction* |
|------|------------|-----------|---------------------|-----------|----------------|-------------------|
|      | Unilateral | Bilateral | Initial or unspecified | Recurrent | | |
| **Inguinal Hernia (into groin)** | | | | | | |
| K40.00 |   | X | X |   |   | X |
| K40.01 |   | X |   | X |   | X |
| K40.10 |   | X | X |   | X |   |
| K40.11 |   | X |   | X | X |   |
| K40.20 |   | X | X |   |   |   |
| K40.21 |   | X |   | X |   |   |
| K40.30 | X |   | X |   |   | X |
| K40.31 | X |   |   | X |   | X |
| K40.40 | X |   | X |   | X |   |
| K40.41 | X |   |   | X | X |   |
| K40.90 | X |   | X |   |   |   |
| K40.91 | X |   |   | X |   |   |
| **Femoral Hernia (into thigh)** | | | | | | |
| K41.00 |   | X | X |   |   | X |
| K41.01 |   | X |   | X |   | X |
| K41.10 |   | X | X |   | X |   |
| K41.11 |   | X |   | X | X |   |
| K41.20 |   | X | X |   |   |   |
| K41.21 |   | X |   | X |   |   |
| K41.30 | X |   | X |   |   | X |
| K41.31 | X |   |   | X |   | X |
| K41.40 | X |   | X |   | X |   |
| K41.41 | X |   |   | X | X |   |
| K41.90 | X |   | X |   |   |   |
| K41.91 | X |   |   | X |   |   |

*If both gangrene and obstruction are documented, list code for gangrene only
If documentation lists strangulated, irreducible or incarcerated, list code for with obstruction

## Coding for Other Hernias

| Code | With Gangrene* | With Obstruction* | Without gangrene or obstruction |
|------|----------------|-------------------|--------------------------------|
| **Umbilical Hernias (into navel)** | | | |
| K42.0 | | X | |
| K42.1 | X | | |
| K42.9 | | | X |
| **Ventral (Incisional) Hernias (into abdominal wall)** | | | |
| K43.0 | | X | |
| K43.1 | X | | |
| K43.2 | | | X |
| **Ventral (parastomal) Hernias (through abdominal opening created surgically)** | | | |
| K43.3 | | X | |
| K43.4 | X | | |
| K43.5 | | | X |
| **Other and Unspecified Ventral Hernias** | | | |
| K43.6 | | X | |
| K43.7 | X | | |
| K43.9 | | | X |
| **Diaphragmatic (Hiatal) Hernias (through diaphragm)** | | | |
| K44.0 | | X | |
| K44.1 | X | | |
| K44.9 | | | X |

*If both gangrene and obstruction are documented, list code for gangrene only
If documentation lists strangulated, irreducible or incarcerated, list code for with obstruction

## Coding for Cholecystitis (Inflammation of *Gallbladder*)

| Code | Type of Cholecystitis | | | | Calculus (Calculi) (Stones) | | |
|------|-------|---------|-------|-------------|----------------------------|--------------------------------|--------------------|
| | Acute | Chronic | Other | Unspecified | Gallbladder (cholelithiasis) | Bile Duct (choledocholithiasis) | With Obstruction |
| K80.00 | X | | | | X | | |
| K80.01 | X | | | | X | | X |
| K80.10 | | X | | | X | | |
| K80.11 | | X | | | X | | X |
| K80.12 | X | X | | | X | | |
| K80.13 | X | X | | | X | | X |
| K80.18 | | | X | | X | | |
| K80.19 | | | X | | X | | X |
| K80.40 | | | | X | | X | |
| K80.41 | | | | X | | X | X |
| K80.42 | X | | | | | X | |
| K80.43 | X | | | | | X | X |
| K80.44 | | X | | | | X | |
| K80.45 | | X | | | | X | X |
| K80.46 | X | X | | | | X | |
| K80.47 | X | X | | | | X | X |
| K80.60 | | | | X | X | X | |
| K80.61 | | | | X | X | X | X |
| K80.62 | X | | | | X | X | |
| K80.63 | X | | | | X | X | X |
| K80.64 | | X | | | X | X | |
| K80.65 | | X | | | X | X | X |
| K80.66 | X | X | | | X | X | |
| K80.67 | X | X | | | X | X | X |
| K81.0 | X | | | | | | |
| K81.1 | | X | | | | | |
| K81.2 | X | X | | | | | |
| K81.9 | | | | X | | | |

## Coding for Cholangitis (Inflammation of *Biliary Tract*)

| Code | Type of Cholangitis | | | | Calculi (Calculus) (Stones) | | |
|------|-------|---------|-------|-------------|----------------------------|--------------------------------|--------------------|
| | Acute | Chronic | Other | Unspecified | Gallbladder (cholelithiasis) | Bile Duct (choledocholithiasis) | With Obstruction |
| K80.30 | | | | X | | X | |
| K80.31 | | | | X | | X | X |
| K80.32 | X | | | | | X | |
| K80.33 | X | | | | | X | X |
| K80.34 | | X | | | | X | |
| K80.35 | | X | | | | X | X |
| K80.36 | X | X | | | | X | |
| K80.37 | X | X | | | | X | X |

## Coding for Calculi Only – No Cholecystitis or Cholangitis

| Code | Calculus (Calculi) (Stones) | | |
| --- | --- | --- | --- |
| | Gallbladder (cholelithiasis) | Bile Duct (choledocholithiasis) | With Obstruction |
| K80.20 | X | | |
| K80.21 | X | | X |
| K80.50 | | X | |
| K80.51 | | X | X |
| K80.70 | X | X | |
| K80.71 | X | X | X |
| K80.80 | X | | |
| K80.81 | X | | X |

# Chapter 12

# Diseases of Skin and Subcutaneous Tissue

These tables are taken from the Official Coding Guidelines, Section I.C.12 (Diseases of the Skin and Subcutaneous Tissue) and Section I.B.14 (General Coding Guidelines, Non-pressure Ulcers and Pressure Ulcer Stages).

Included in this chapter are these tables:

1) Coding Pressure Ulcers
2) Pressure Ulcer Stages
3) Coding Non-Pressure Ulcers
4) Non-Pressure Ulcers Depths
5) Documentation for Pressure and Non-Pressure Ulcers
6) Coding Cellulitis

## Coding Pressure Ulcers*

| Description/Number of Pressure Ulcer(s) | Principal Diagnosis | Additional Diagnoses |
| --- | --- | --- |
| One ulcer | Any associated gangrene if documented – I96 | Site and stage of ulcer – from category L89 |
| Bilateral ulcers – same or different stages | Any associated gangrene if documented – I96 | Separate codes for each site (right and left) or stage – from category L89 |
| Multiple ulcers – different sites | Any associated gangrene if documented – I96 | Separate codes for each ulcer – from category L89 |
| Healing ulcer | Any associated gangrene if documented – I96 | Site and stage of ulcer as currently documented – from category L89 |
| Healed ulcer | Do **NOT** code | Do not code |
| Ulcer at one site changes stage during hospitalization | Any associated gangrene if documented – I96 | List one code for stage at admission and Another code for highest stage reported during admission from category L89 |

*List as many codes as needed to fully describe site and stage of all pressure ulcers documented.

If patient has pressure ulcer at admission but it has healed at discharge, assign code for site and stage of pressure ulcer at time of admission

## Pressure Ulcer Stages

| Stage | Definition |
|---|---|
| Stage 1 | Skin changes limited to persistent focal edema (swelling confined to small area) |
| Stage 2 | Abrasion, blister, partial thickness skin loss involving epidermis and/or dermis |
| Stage 3 | Full thickness skin loss involving damage or necrosis of subcutaneous tissue |
| Stage 4 | Necrosis of soft tissues through to underlying muscle, tendon or bone |
| Unstageable | Stage cannot be clinically determined. This may be because the ulcer is:<br>1) Covered by eschar (scab) OR<br>2) Has been treated with a skin or muscle graft (and therefore cannot be viewed directly) OR<br>3) Documented as a deep tissue injury not due to trauma. |
| Unspecified | Provider did not list sufficient documentation to select stage |

## Coding Non-Pressure Ulcers of Skin

| Type of Ulcer | Principal Diagnosis | Secondary Diagnoses |
|---|---|---|
| Chronic ulcer of lower limb | Any associated underlying condition<br>Associated gangrene if documented | Non-pressure chronic ulcer of lower limb – L97 |
| Chronic ulcer of other sites | Code from L98 according to ulcer site | |
| Diabetic ulcer | Code for type of diabetes – E08.62x, E09.62x, E10.62x, E11.62x, or E13.62x | Code for site of ulcer – L97 or L98 |

## Non-Pressure Ulcer Depths

| Description of Depth | 6th Digits |
|---|---|
| Limited to breakdown of skin | 1 |
| With fat layer exposed | 2 |
| With necrosis of muscle | 3 |
| With necrosis of bone | 4 |
| Unspecified | 9 |

## Documentation of Pressure and Non-Pressure Ulcers

| Codes | Coding Guidelines |
|---|---|
| Non-Pressure Ulcers | Presence of ulcer must be documented by physician<br>Depth of ulcer may be documented by nonphysician providers (dietician or nurse)<br>If documentation from providers is conflicting, query physician |
| Pressure ulcers | Presence of ulcer must be documented by physician<br>Stage of ulcer may be documented by nonphysician provider (dietician or nurse)<br>If documentation from providers is conflicting, query physician |

# Coding Cellulitis

| Condition | Coding Guidelines |
| --- | --- |
| Cellulitis with acute lymphangitis | List code for cellulitis<br>Then code for infection (B95-B96) |
| Cellulitis with abscess | List code for cellulitis<br>Then code for infection (B95-B96) |
| Cellulitis with superficial injury | List codes for both conditions.<br>Sequencing depends on circumstances of visit |
| Cellulitis with open wound | List code for complicated open wound and code for cellulitis.<br>Sequencing depends on circumstances of visit |
| Cellulitis in operative wound | Code first infection following procedure (T81.4)<br>Then code cellulitis (L03-)<br>Then code for infection (B95-B96) |
| Cellulitis with burn | List codes for both conditions.<br>Sequencing depends on circumstances of visit |
| Cellulitis with frostbite | List codes for both conditions.<br>Sequencing depends on circumstances of visit |
| Cellulitis with gangrene | List code for gangrene only (I96) |
| Cellulitis with chronic skin ulcer | List codes for both conditions.<br>Sequencing depends on circumstances of visit |

# Chapter 13

# Diseases of the Musculoskeletal System and Connective Tissue

These tables are taken from the Official Coding Guidelines, Section I.C.13 (Diseases of the Musculoskeletal System and Connective Tissue).

Included in this chapter are these tables:

1) Coding Conditions in Bones, Joints or Muscles
2) Pathological Fractures – 7th digits
3) Coding Osteoporosis

## Coding Conditions in Bones, Joints, or Muscles

| Condition involves - | Coding Guidelines | Examples |
|---|---|---|
| **Conditions involve multiple sites (bones, joints or muscles)** | | |
| Bilateral sites | List separate codes for right and left or Bilateral code if available | Pain in both wrists (no bilateral codes available) M25.531 – right wrist M25.532 – left wrist |
| Multiple specific sites | List one code for multiple sites if available OR | M89.571 - Osteolysis, right ankle and foot |
| Multiple specific sites | List separate codes for each site | M46.24 – Osteomyelitis, thoracic region M46.26 – Osteomyelitis, lumbar region |
| Multiple nonspecific sites | List one code for multiple sites | M06.09 - Rheumatoid arthritis without rheumatoid factors, multiple sites |
| **Other Guidelines** | | |
| Portion of a bone at a joint | List code for bone, not joint | Idiopathic avascular necrosis of femoral head of left hip joint – List code for bone (M87.052) not hip joint |
| Chronic condition due to previous injury or trauma | List code from chapter 13 (musculoskeletal system) | Old bucket handle tear of right medial meniscus – List code for old tear or injury (M23.203) |
| Recurrent condition | List code from chapter 13 (musculoskeletal system) | Recurrent dislocation of patella – List code for recurrent condition (M22.01) |
| Current, acute injury | List code from chapter 19 (Injuries) | Bucket handle tear of right medial meniscus – List code for current injury (S83.211A) |
| Complication of surgical treatment of fracture | List code for complication and code for fracture | During healing or recovery phase of treatment Circumstances of admission determine which code is listed first |
| Documentation is unclear as to whether code is due to injury or disease condition | Query provider | |

## Pathological Fractures – 7$^{th}$ Digits*

| 7$^{th}$ Digit | Encounter | Definition | Examples |
|---|---|---|---|
| A | Initial | Patient receiving active treatment | Surgical treatment<br>ER encounter<br>Evaluation and continuing treatment by same or new physician |
| D | Subsequent | Active treatment completed<br>Patient seen for routine care during healing or recovery phase | Cast change or removal<br>X-ray to check healing status of fracture<br>Removal of external or internal fixation device<br>Medication adjustment<br>Other aftercare |
| G | Subsequent | Active treatment completed<br>Delayed healing | Healing process taking longer than usual. May be due to swelling, infection, or nerve damage |
| K | Subsequent | Active treatment completed<br>Nonunion | Fracture fragments failed to properly unite |
| P | Subsequent | Active treatment completed<br>Malunion | Fracture fragments failed to properly align |
| S | Sequela | Patient seen for treatment of complication or conditions that arose as a direct result of injury | Scar<br>Abnormality in gait due to previous injury |

Do not list aftercare Z codes if a 7$^{th}$ digit for subsequent encounter is available.

*Not all fracture codes include all these possible digits.

## Coding Osteoporosis

| Osteoporosis due to - | Osteoporosis with current pathological fracture* | Osteoporosis without current pathological fracture | |
|---|---|---|---|
| | | No history of pathological fracture | History of pathological fracture |
| Age (postmenopausal) | Category M80 | Category M81 | Code first M81<br>Code also Z87.310 |
| Neoplasm | Subcategory M84.5- | Category M81 | Code first M81<br>Code also Z87.311 |
| Other conditions | Subcategory M84.6- | Category M81 | Code first M81<br>Code also Z87.311 |

*Fracture codes are for site of <u>fracture</u>, not site of the <u>osteoporosis</u>

Be sure to use 7$^{th}$ digits!

# Chapter 14

# Diseases of Genitourinary System

These tables are taken from the Official Coding Guidelines: Section I.C.1 (Certain Infectious and Parasitic Diseases), Section I.C.9 (Diseases of Circulatory System); Section I.C.14 (Diseases of Genitourinary System); and Section 1.C.21 (Factors Influencing Health Status and Contact with Health Services).

Included in this chapter are these tables:

1) Coding for Chronic Kidney Disease (CKD)
2) Coding for Incontinence
3) Coding for Urinary Tract Infections
4) Z Codes for Reproductive Health Services

## Coding for Chronic Kidney Disease (CKD)

| Documentation Indicates - | Principal Diagnosis | Secondary Diagnoses | Comments |
|---|---|---|---|
| Hypertension and CKD | Category I12 (hypertensive CKD) | Category N18 (CKD) Category N17 (renal failure) if documented | Assume a relationship between hypertension and CKD |
| Hypertension, heart disease and CKD | Category I13 (hypertensive heart and CKD) | Category N18 (CKD) Category I50 (heart failure) if documented | Assume a relationship between hypertension, heart disease and CKD |
| Stage of CKD and end stage renal disease | N18.6 (end stage renal disease) | | Do **NOT** list code for stage of CKD |
| CKD with other conditions | Code separately for CKD (N18) and other conditions Circumstances of admission determine which code is listed first | | |
| CKD with previous kidney transplant | Category N18 | Z94.0 – history of kidney transplant | Do **NOT** assume that condition is complication of transplant |
| Complication due to previous kidney transplant* | T86.1- (complication of kidney transplant) | Specific complication | Condition must be documented as due to complication of transplant |

*Complication of kidney transplant – patient may still have some form of CKD after transplant because transplant did not complete restore kidney function. This is not a complication unless documented as such by the provider.

## Coding for Incontinence

| Type of Incontinence | Definition | Codes |
|---|---|---|
| Stress | Patient voids involuntarily when laughing, coughing, etc. | N39.3 Code also overactive bladder if documented (N32.81) |
| Urge | Patient cannot control urge to urinate | N39.41 Code also overactive bladder if documented (N32.81) |
| Incontinence without sensory awareness | Patient experiences reduced signals of need to urinate | N39.42 Code also overactive bladder if documented (N32.81) |
| Post-void dribbling | Patient experiences involuntary discharge of residual urine after voiding | N39.43 Code also overactive bladder if documented (N32.81) |
| Nocturnal enuresis | Patient needs to get up at night to urinate | N39.44 Code also overactive bladder if documented (N32.81) |
| Continuous leakage | Patient has constant leaking of urine | N39.45 Code also overactive bladder if documented (N32.81) |
| Mixed incontinence | Patient experience both urge and stress incontinence | N39.46 Code also overactive bladder if documented (N32.81) |
| Overflow leakage | Patient experiences incontinence due to weakened bladder muscles | N39.490 Code also overactive bladder if documented (N32.81) |
| Functional incontinence | Patient has physical impairment (physical condition) that prevents him/her from reaching toilet in time | R39.81 |
| Incontinence with cognitive impairment | Patient has cognitive impairment (mental condition) that interferes with recognition of need to urinate | R39.81 |
| Unspecified Enuresis NOS | Not enough documentation to select another more specific code. Enuresis is defined as bedwetting. | R32 |
| Incontinence of nonorganic origin | Patient (usually child or adolescent) has behavioral or emotional disorders that result in incontinence | F98.0 |

## Coding for Urinary Tract Infections

| Condition | Codes | Guidelines |
|---|---|---|
| Urinary tract infection, site unspecified (NOS) | N39.0 | List also code B95-B97 to indicate bacteria or virus causing infection |
| Urinary tract infection, site specified | | |
|    Bladder (cystitis) | N30- | List also code B95-B97 to indicate bacteria or virus causing infection |
|    Kidney (tubulo-interstitial nephritis) | N10 - N12 | List also code B95-B97 to indicate bacteria or virus causing infection |
|    Urethra (urethritis) | N34- | List also code B95-B97 to indicate bacteria or virus causing infection |
| Urosepsis | NO CODE | This is a nonspecific term without a diagnosis code. Query physician for more information to select a specific code |

## Z Codes for Reproductive Health Services

| Code | | Coding Guidelines |
|---|---|---|
| Z30 | Encounter for contraceptive management | Patient is trying NOT to become pregnant |
| Z31 | Encounter for procreative management | Patient is trying to become pregnant |
| Z32.0- | Encounter for pregnancy test | 5th digit indicates results - unknown, positive or negative |

# Chapter 15

# Pregnancy, Childbirth and the Puerperium

These tables are taken from the Official Coding Guidelines, Section I.C.9 (Diseases of Circulatory System); Section I.C.15 (Pregnancy, Childbirth and the Puerperium); Section I.C.19.e (Injury, Poisoning, and Certain Other Consequences of External Causes, Poisoning, Underdosing and Toxic Effects), Section I.C.19.f (Injury, Poisoning, and Certain Other Consequences of External Causes, Adult and Child Abuse); and Section 1.C.21.c.11) (Factors Influencing Health Status and Contact with Health Services, Encounters for Obstetrical and Reproductive Services).

Included in this chapter are these tables:

1) Trimester Definitions
2) Trimester Guidelines
3) Digits for Fetus
4) Conditions that May Be Maternal or Fetal Conditions
5) Coding Guidelines Related to Episode of Care
6) Coding Hypertension-related Conditions in Pregnancy
7) Coding Diabetes in Pregnancy
8) Guidelines for Other Specific Conditions Complicating Pregnancy, Childbirth and the puerperium
9) Coding for Pregnancy with Abortive Outcomes
10) Z Codes for Obstetrical Services

## Trimester Definitions

| Encounter | Definition |
|---|---|
| 1st trimester | Less than 14 weeks, 0 days |
| 2nd trimester | 14 weeks 0 days to less than 28 weeks, 0 days |
| 3rd trimester | 28 weeks 0 days until delivery |
| Unspecified trimester | Documentation does not indicate weeks gestation |
| Childbirth | Patient delivered during this admission |
| Puerperium | Patient delivered during previous admission |

Zero days means after the 7th day of the week. For example:
1. Documentation indicates patient is 14 weeks and 3 days pregnant, use a digit for 2nd trimester (3 days into 2nd trimester).
2. Documentation indicates patient is 13 weeks and 6 days, use digit of 1st trimester (one day short of 2nd trimester minimum of 14 weeks).

# Trimester Guidelines

| Circumstances | Coding Guidelines |
|---|---|
| Patient admitted for acute complication during one trimester; remains hospitalized into next trimester | Use digit for trimester when patient was admitted |
| Patient developed complication prior to admission or encounter | Use digit for trimester when admitted or first seen |
| Delivery occurs during current admission | Use digit for childbirth if available |
| Condition includes trimester digits for only some trimesters, not all three | This indicates that condition only occurs during the trimesters for which digits are available |
| Code does not include trimester digits | This indicates that the condition always occurs in a specific trimester or trimester is not applicable |
| Unspecified trimester | Trimester not documented by provider. Rarely used in inpatient admissions. |

Some codes in this chapter use a digit to indicate which fetus is involved for cases of pregnancy with multiple fetuses. These digits are used to indicate which fetus has condition, not the total number of fetuses in the pregnancy. List also code from O30 (multiple gestation) to indicate total number of fetuses. Seventh digits for fetus are as follows:

## Digits for Fetus

| Definition | 7th Digit |
|---|---|
| Only one fetus | 0 |
| No documentation as to which fetus affected | 0 |
| Physician cannot determine which fetus is affected | 0 |
| Multiple fetuses – condition in fetus 1 | 1 |
| Multiple fetuses – condition in fetus 2 | 2 |
| Multiple fetuses – condition in fetus 3 | 3 |
| Multiple fetuses – condition in fetus 4 | 4 |
| Multiple fetuses – condition in fetus 5 | 5 |
| Multiple fetuses – condition in fetus 6 or more | 9 |

Most codes in this chapter refer to conditions in the mother that complicate her care during pregnancy. Other codes, however, refer to conditions in the fetus that complicate care for the mother.

Some conditions can be coded as maternal problems or fetal problems, depending on the circumstances. Even if the fetus has the condition, it is the mother who is the patient. Following are some examples:

## Conditions that May Be Maternal or Fetal Conditions*

| Condition | Maternal Condition* | Fetus damaged by maternal condition |
|---|---|---|
| Viral disease | O98.5- | O35.3- |
| Use of alcohol | O99.31- | O35.4- |
| Use of drugs | O99.32- | O35.5- |
| Retained intrauterine device | O26.3- | O35.7- |

These codes are listed only when the fetal condition is modifying the management of the pregnant patient (requiring diagnostic studies, additional observation, special care or termination of the pregnancy).

# Coding Guidelines Related to Episode of Care

| Reason for Admission | Definitions | Coding Guidelines |
|---|---|---|
| **Antepartum – No Delivery This Episode of Care** | | |
| Routine prenatal visit | Routine outpatient visit with no complications | List first code Z34<br>Do **NOT** list any codes from chapter 15 |
| Prenatal visit for high risk patient | Prenatal visit with patient who had:<br>1) Complication during previous pregnancy (such as pre-term labor) OR<br>2) Has high risk factor in this pregnancy (such as elderly primigravida) | List first code from O09 category<br>List other codes from chapter 15 as appropriate |
| Complication <u>related</u> to pregnancy | Patient admitted for condition that is due to or related to her pregnancy | List complication code from chapter 15<br>If more than one condition treated or monitored, any may be listed first |
| Condition <u>unrelated</u> to pregnancy | Patient admitted for condition that is not due to or related to her pregnancy | Provider must document condition is unrelated<br>List first code for unrelated condition<br>Then list code Z33.1 (pregnancy incidental) |
| **Delivery This Episode of Care** | | |
| Uncomplicated delivery | Delivery is documented as (all must apply):<br>1) Spontaneous 6) Minimal or no assistance<br>2) Cephalic<br>3) Vaginal 7) With or without episiotomy<br>4) Full-term<br>5) Single, live born infant 8) No fetal manipulation or instrumentation | List first code O80<br>Do **NOT** list other codes from chapter 15.<br>May list codes from other chapters if appropriate<br>Patient may have had complication at some point in pregnancy, but none are present at time of admission for delivery<br>Only outcome of delivery code listed with O80 is Z37.0 |
| Vaginal delivery | Vaginal delivery during this hospitalization | List first main circumstance or complication of delivery<br>If multiple conditions resulted in admission, list first one most related to delivery |
| Cesarean delivery | Admitted for condition <u>related</u> to cesarean delivery | List first code for condition related to cesarean delivery<br>If multiple conditions resulted in admission, list first one most related to delivery |
| | Admitted for condition <u>unrelated</u> to cesarean delivery; cesarean during this admission | List first code for condition related to admission |
| Outcome of delivery | Must be listed on maternal record when delivery occurred during the admission | List first code related to delivery<br>Then list code Z37-<br>Do not list on subsequent records or newborn records - Once in a lifetime code |

**CONTINUED ON NEXT PAGE**

# Coding Guidelines Related to Episode of Care (continued)

| Reason for Admission | Definitions | Coding Guidelines |
|---|---|---|
| **Postpartum Care – Period from delivery to 6 weeks after delivery\*** | | |
| Routine postpartum care following delivery outside hospital | Routine care with no complications | List first code Z39.0 |
| Other routine postpartum care | Routine care with no complications. Delivery occurred during previous encounter | List first code Z39.1 or Z39.2 |
| Complication related to pregnancy | Provider must document condition is related | Code first specific condition. Then list code from chapter 15 |
| Puerperal sepsis | Patient develops sepsis after delivery | List first code from O85-. Then list: 1) Code B95-B96 for bacteria or virus that caused sepsis 2) Code R65.2 (if severe sepsis) and 3) Code for organ dysfunction if appropriate. Do **NOT** list codes A40 or (streptococcal sepsis) or A41 (other sepsis) |
| **Sequelae** | | |
| Sequelae | Initial. treated complication of a pregnancy develops sequelae requiring care or treatment. | Code first specific condition and then O94. Use any time after postpartum period |

\*If complication is documented as related to the pregnancy but occurs after 6 weeks postpartum, code for complication of pregnancy.

# Coding Hypertension-Related Conditions in Pregnancy

| Code | | Digits | Additional Diagnoses |
|---|---|---|---|
| **Pre-existing Hypertension (Patient had hypertension *before* becoming pregnant)** | | | |
| O10.0- | Essential hypertension | Digits for trimesters 1-3, childbirth and puerperium | - |
| O10.1- | Hypertension with heart disease | Digits for trimesters 1-3, childbirth and puerperium | Code from category I11 |
| O10.2- | Hypertension with chronic kidney disease | Digits for trimesters 1-3, childbirth and puerperium | Code from category I12 |
| O10.3- | Hypertension with heart and chronic kidney disease | Digits for trimesters 1-3, childbirth and puerperium | Code from Category I13 |
| O10.4- | Secondary hypertension | Digits for trimesters 1-3, childbirth and puerperium | Code from Category I15 |
| O10.90 | Unspecified hypertension | Digits for trimesters 1-3, childbirth and puerperium | - |
| O11- | Hypertension with pre-eclampsia | Digits for trimesters 1-3 No digits for childbirth or puerperium | Code from Category O10 |
| **Gestational Conditions (Patient developed conditions *after* becoming pregnant)** | | | |
| O12.0- | Edema without hypertension | Digits for trimesters 1-3 No digits for childbirth or puerperium | - |
| O12.1- | Proteinuria without hypertension | Digits for trimesters 1-3 No digits for childbirth or puerperium | - |
| O12.2- | Edema with proteinuria | Digits for trimesters 1-3 No digits for childbirth or puerperium | - |
| O13- | Hypertension without significant proteinuria | Digits for trimesters1-3 No digits for childbirth or puerperium | - |
| O14- | Pre-eclampsia | Digits for trimesters 2-3 only No digits for childbirth or puerperium | - |
| O15- | Eclampsia | Digits for trimesters 2-3 only No digits for childbirth or puerperium | - |
| **Hypertension unspecified as to whether Pre-existing or Gestational** | | | |
| O16- | Unspecified maternal hypertension | Digits for trimesters 1-3 No digits for childbirth or puerperium | - |

Note that pre-eclampsia and eclampsia include only digits for 2nd and 3rd trimester since the condition does not appear until the 2nd trimester.

Note also that gestational and unspecified hypertension do not include digits for childbirth or puerperium

## Coding Diabetes in Pregnancy

| Code | | Digits | Additional Diagnoses |
|---|---|---|---|
| **Pre-existing Diabetes (Patient had diabetes *before* becoming pregnant)** | | | |
| O24.0- | Type 1 diabetes | Digits for trimesters 1-3, childbirth and puerperium | Code from category E10 |
| O24.1- | Type 2 diabetes | Digits for trimesters 1-3, childbirth and puerperium | Code from category E11 Code Z79.4 if appropriate |
| O24.3- | Unspecified diabetes | Digits for trimesters 1-3, childbirth and puerperium | Code from category E11 Code Z79.4 if appropriate |
| O24.8- | Other pre-existing diabetes | Digits for trimesters 1-3, childbirth and puerperium | Code from category E08, E09 or E13 Code Z79.4 if appropriate |
| **Gestational (Patient developed diabetes *after* becoming pregnant)\*** | | | |
| O24.41- | Diabetes in pregnancy | No specific digits for trimesters Digits indicate method used to control diabetes (diet, insulin or unspecified) | Do **NOT** list code Z79.4 |
| O24.42- | Diabetes in childbirth | No specific digits for trimesters Digits indicate method used to control diabetes (diet, insulin or unspecified) | Do **NOT** list code Z79.4 |
| O24.43- | Diabetes in puerperium | No specific digits for trimesters Digits indicate method used to control diabetes (diet, insulin or unspecified) | Do **NOT** list code Z79.4 |
| O99.81- | Abnormal glucose | No specific digits for trimester Digits for pregnancy, childbirth and puerperium | |
| **Diabetes Unspecified as Pre-existing or Gestational** | | | |
| O24.9- | Unspecified diabetes | Digits for trimesters 1-3, childbirth and puerperium | Code Z79.4 if appropriate |

\*If patient treated with both oral medications and insulin, list only the code for insulin-controlled.

\*If patient treated with diet and oral hypoglycemic drugs, list only the code for oral hypoglycemic drugs.

# Guidelines for Other Specific Conditions Complicating Pregnancy, Childbirth and Puerperium

| Code | Condition | Digits | Coding Guidelines |
|------|-----------|--------|-------------------|
| O90.3- | Cardiomyopathy - developed <u>during</u> pregnancy | No digits for trimester, childbirth or puerperium | May be diagnosed in 3<sup>rd</sup> trimester but continue into months after delivery |
| O99.4- | Cardiomyopathy – developed <u>before</u> pregnancy | Digits for trimesters 1-3. Childbirth and puerperium | |
| O9A.3-<br>O9A.5- | Abuse in pregnant patient | Digits for trimesters 1-3, childbirth and puerperium | List first O9A.3-O9A.5<br>Then list code for specific injury if documented<br>Then list code for perpetrator (Y07-) |
| O35- | In utero surgery | No digits for trimester, childbirth or puerperium<br>Digits for which fetus | List first O35-<br>Do **NOT** list code from chapter 16 (perinatal conditions) |
| O98.7- | HIV/AIDS | Digits for trimesters 1-3, childbirth and puerperium | List first O98.7-<br>Then HIV/AIDS code B20 or Z21<br>Then code for any HIV related conditions if documented |
| O85- | Puerperal sepsis | No digits for trimester, childbirth or puerperium | List first O85-<br>Then list:<br>4) Code B95-B96 for bacteria or virus that caused sepsis<br>5) Code R65.2 (if severe sepsis) and<br>6) Code for organ dysfunction if appropriate<br>Do **NOT** list codes A40 or (streptococcal sepsis) or A41 (other sepsis) |
| O99.31- | Alcohol use | Digits for trimesters 1-3 childbirth and puerperium | List first O99.31-<br>Then list code F10 alcohol related disorders |
| O99.32- | Drug use | Digits for trimesters 1-3, Childbirth and puerperium | List first O99.32-<br>Then list code F11-F16 and F18-F19 |
| O99.33- | Tobacco use (any type) | Digits for trimesters 1-3, childbirth and puerperium | List first O99.33-<br>Then list code F17 to indicate type of tobacco |
| O9A.2- | Poisoning, toxic effects and underdosing | Digits for trimester 1-3, childbirth and puerperium | List first O9A.2<br>Then list:<br>1) Code for poisoning, adverse effect, toxic effect or underdosing<br>2) Any resulting conditions |

# Codes for Pregnancy with Abortive Outcomes

| Codes | | Additional Digits | Definitions/Guidelines |
|---|---|---|---|
| **Abnormal Products of Conception** | | | |
| O00 | Ectopic pregnancy | 4th digits – location | Fertilized egg implants outside of uterus |
| O01 | Hydatidiform mole | 4th digits - type | Early placenta develops into mass of cysts<br>List additional code from category O08 to indicate associated complication |
| O02 | Other abnormal products of conception | 4th digits - type | Includes codes for blighted ovum and missed abortion<br>List additional code from category O08 to indicate associated complication |
| O08* | Complications following ectopic and molar pregnancy | 4th or 5th digits - specific complications | List codes from category O08 with codes from O00 and O01 to report specific complications. |
| **Spontaneous Abortion (Miscarriage; Loss of Fetus due to Natural Causes)** | | | |
| O03 | Spontaneous abortion (miscarriage) | 5th digits – specific complication | Fetal loss without physician intervention |
| | Incomplete spontaneous abortion | O03.0-O03.4<br>5th digits – specific complication | Patient had miscarriage but not all products of conception are expelled |
| | Complete or unspecified spontaneous abortion | O03.5-O03.9– 5th digits - complete or spontaneous abortion | All products of conception are expelled |
| | Complete spontaneous abortion.<br>Patient readmitted due to retained products of conception | O03.0-O03.4<br>Incomplete abortion for second encounter | This guideline applies even if first encounter was coded as complete abortion |
| **Induced Abortions – Loss of Fetus due to Physician Intervention** | | | |
| O04 | Induced termination of pregnancy | 4th or 5th digits - specific complications | List this code if complication of abortion documented |
| O07* | Failed attempted termination of pregnancy | 4th or 5th digits - specific complications | List this code if complication of abortion documented.<br>If liveborn fetus, list also code Z37 |
| Z33.2 | Encounter for elective termination of pregnancy | No additional digits | Always listed first<br>List this code if no complications of abortion documented<br>If Liveborn fetus, list also code Z37 |

*If appropriate, list an additional code from chapter 15 with codes from O07 and O08 to indicate complications of the pregnancy

# Z Codes for Obstetrical Services

| Code | | Coding Guidelines |
|------|------|-------------------|
| Z03.7- | Encounter for suspected maternal and fetal conditions ruled out | List additional codes only if reporting conditions unrelated to suspected condition.<br>Circumstances of admission determine which code is listed first<br>Do **NOT** list this code if condition confirmed or signs/symptoms are documented. See codes O35, O36, )40 and O41<br>For encounters for antenatal screening, see code Z36 |
| Z33.1 | Pregnancy incidental | Patient seen for condition documented as unrelated to pregnancy<br>List first unrelated condition<br>Then list this code |
| Z33.2 | Encounter for elective termination of pregnancy | Always listed first.<br>Listed for uncomplicated termination<br>Then list codes from chapter 15 if appropriate |
| Z34- | Encounter for supervision of normal pregnancy | Always listed first<br>Listed for routine antepartum visit with no complications<br>Do **NOT** list with any codes from chapter 15 |
| Z36 | Encounter for antenatal screening of mother | List this code for routine screening<br>Mother and fetus have no signs or symptoms of abnormal condition |
| Z3A | Weeks of gestation | List on all maternal records if documented<br>If complication present at admission, list code for weeks at date of admission<br>If complication develops after admission, list code for weeks when complication developed<br>Do **NOT** use this code for pregnancies with abortive outcomes, elective termination of pregnancy, or postpartum conditions |
| Z37 | Outcome of delivery | Never listed first<br>List on maternal record when delivery occurred during this admission<br>Do **NOT** list on newborn record |
| Z76.81 | Counseling for expectant mother | List for prebirth visit with potential pediatrician |
| O35, O36, O40, or O41 | Observation and testing for abnormal condition in fetus. Abnormal condition or symptoms found | Do **NOT** list observation code (Z03.7) |

# Chapter 16

# Certain Conditions Originating in the Perinatal Period

These tables are taken from the Official Coding Guidelines, Section I.C.16 (Certain Conditions Originating in the Perinatal Period) and Section 1.C.21.c.12) (Factors Influencing Health Status and Contact with Health Services, Newborns and Infants).

Included in this chapter are these tables:

1) General Coding Guidelines
2) Coding Guidelines for Specific Conditions
3) Examples of Conditions that May Be Maternal, Fetal or Newborn Conditions
4) Examples of Conditions that May Be Perinatal or Acquired
5) Z codes for Conditions in the Newborn

## General Coding Guidelines

| Reason for Admission | Coding Guidelines |
|---|---|
| Significant perinatal condition | List code for any condition that:<br>1) Requires clinical evaluation<br>2) Requires therapeutic treatment<br>3) Requires diagnostic procedures<br>4) Prolongs length of stay<br>5) Requires increased nursing care and/or monitoring<br>6) Has implications for future health care needs |
| Reason for admission is perinatal condition | List first perinatal condition<br>Then list other conditions as appropriate |
| Birth admission (newborn delivered this admission) | List first Z38 - List only once for birth admission<br>Then codes from chapter 16 or other chapters as appropriate |
| Condition may or may not be due to birth process | If documentation unclear, list a code for due to birth process |
| Perinatal condition in older patient | Condition still present - List perinatal code |
| Signs and symptoms without definitive diagnosis | List codes from chapter 18 |

# Coding Guidelines for Specific Conditions

| Code | Conditions | Coding Guidelines |
|---|---|---|
| PO5- | Slow fetal growth and fetal malnutrition | Must be documented by provider<br>Do **NOT** code with PO7 |
| P07- | Short gestation and low birth weight | Must be documented by provider<br>List this code for child or adult who:<br>    a) Was born prematurely or had low birth weight AND<br>    b) Condition is still affecting patient's current health status<br>Do **NOT** code with PO5 |
| PO7.0-P07.2 | Birth weight | If both birth weight and prematurity are documented:<br>List first code PO7.0-PO7.2 |
| P07.3- | Prematurity | Then list code P07.3- |
| P36- | Bacterial sepsis of newborn | Includes congenital sepsis<br>If unclear whether sepsis is congenital or community-acquired, list code for congenital<br>4$^{th}$ digit indicates bacteria or virus that caused sepsis<br>For code P36.8 – list additional code from B95-B96<br>If severe sepsis, list also code R65.2- and codes for any associated organ dysfunctions if appropriate |
| P95 | Stillborn | Listed only in institutions that maintain separate records for stillbirths<br>Do **NOT** list any other code with this one<br>Do **NOT** list on maternal record. List Z37.1 instead |

Some conditions have different codes depending on whether the condition is found in the pregnant mother, the fetus or newborn. Following are some examples:

## Examples of Conditions that May Be Maternal, Fetal or Newborn Conditions

| Condition | Maternal condition* | Fetus damaged by maternal condition* | Newborn damaged by maternal condition** |
|---|---|---|---|
| Viral disease | O98.5- | O35.3- | P00.2 |
| Use of alcohol | O99.31- | O35.4- | P04.3 |
| Use of drugs | O99.32- | O35.5- | P04.4- |
| Retained intrauterine device | O99.33- | O35.7- | P04.2 |

*Never list maternal code on newborn's medical record.

**Never list newborn code on mother's medical record.

Some conditions have different codes indicating whether the condition is perinatal or acquired. Following are some examples:

## Examples of Conditions that May Be Perinatal or Acquired

| Condition | Perinatal Code | Acquired Code |
|---|---|---|
| Bradycardia | P29.12 | R00.1 |
| Interstitial emphysema | P25.0 | J98.2 |
| Tachypnea | P22.1 | R06.82 |
| Hematemesis | P54.0 | K92.0 |

## Z Codes for Conditions in the Newborn

| Code | | Coding Guidelines |
|---|---|---|
| Z00.1- | Encounter for routine child health exam | Child is under 29 days old<br>If abnormal findings:<br>List first Z00.1- code<br>Then list code for any findings |
| Z05 | Observation and evaluation of newborns and infants for suspected condition ruled out | Healthy newborn is evaluated for a suspected condition but after study the condition is not found. May be listed as principal/first-listed diagnosis in cases when Z38 does not apply.<br>Do **NOT** use this code if the newborn has signs or symptoms of a suspected problem. Use a code for the sign or symptom instead. |
| Z38 | Liveborn infants according to place of birth and type of delivery | Always listed first on newborn record<br>Then list Z05 if appropriate<br>Do **NOT** list on maternal record |

# Chapter 17

# Congenital Malformations, Deformations,

# and Chromosomal Abnormalities

These tables are taken from the Official Coding Guidelines, Section I.C.17 (Congenital Malformations, Deformations, and Chromosomal Abnormalities).

Included in this chapter are these tables:

1) General Coding Guidelines
2) Examples of Conditions that May Be Maternal, Fetal, Perinatal or Congenital

## General Coding Guidelines

| Circumstances/Conditions | Coding Guidelines |
|---|---|
| Sequencing | Circumstances of admission determine which code is listed first |
| Condition is integral to congenital anomaly/syndrome | Do **NOT** code condition separately.<br>Example: Tetralogy of Fallot<br>List code Q21.3. Do not list additional codes for associated septal defect or pulmonary stenosis. |
| Condition is NOT integral to congenital anomaly/syndrome | Code conditions separately.<br>Example: Cockayne's Syndrome with mental retardation, retinal atrophy and microcephaly<br>List codes Q87.1, H35.89, F79, and Q02 |
| Condition diagnosed during birth admission | Code first Z38<br>Then list code for congenital condition |
| Condition diagnosed at birth; patient now older | Condition still present - List perinatal code<br>Condition successfully treated – List history code |
| Condition was present at birth but not diagnosed until patient is older | List congenital code |

Some conditions can be coded as maternal problems, fetal problems, or congenital problems depending on the circumstances.  Following are some examples:

## Examples of Conditions that May Be Maternal, Fetal, Perinatal or Congenital

| Diagnoses | Maternal condition | Fetal condition | Perinatal Condition | Congenital condition |
|---|---|---|---|---|
| Use of alcohol | O99.31- | O35.4 | P04.3 | Q86.0* |
| Conjoined twins | | O30.02- | | Q89.4 |
| Chromosomal abnormality | | O35.1- | | Q90-Q99 |

*Q86.0 – Fetal alcohol syndrome

# Chapter 18

## Symptoms, Signs, and Abnormal Clinical and Laboratory Findings, Not Elsewhere Classified

These tables are taken from the Official Coding Guidelines I.C.1 (Certain Infectious and Parasitic Diseases); I.C.18 (Symptoms, Signs and Abnormal Clinical and Laboratory Findings, Not Elsewhere Classified); General Guidelines I.B.4 (Signs and Symptoms), Section II (Selection of Principal Diagnosis); Section III (Reporting Additional Diagnoses); and Section IV (Diagnostic Coding and Reporting Guidelines for Outpatient Services).

Included in this chapter are these tables:

1) General Coding Guidelines
2) Coma scale
3) NIH Stroke Scale
4) Coding Sepsis/Severe Sepsis
5) Guidelines for Other Specific Conditions

### General Coding Guidelines

| Documented conditions | Principal diagnosis | Comments |
|---|---|---|
| Patient seen for symptoms; Definitive diagnosis NOT known by end of encounter | Symptom | |
| Definitive diagnosis known; Symptoms are related to definitive diagnosis | Definitive diagnosis | Do **NOT** list code for signs and symptoms |
| Definitive diagnosis known; Symptoms are NOT related to definitive diagnosis | Definitive diagnosis | List also codes for signs and symptoms |
| Combination codes – include both definitive diagnosis and symptom | Combination code only | Do **NOT** code separately for symptom For example: K50.011 – Crohn's disease with rectal bleeding. Do **NOT** list separate code for bleeding |
| INPATIENT discharged with condition documented as probable, suspected, likely, questionable, possible, or still to be ruled out | Suspected condition as if confirmed | |
| OUTPATIENT discharged with condition documented as probable, suspected, likely, questionable, possible, or still to be ruled out | Symptoms | Do **NOT** code suspected condition as if confirmed |

## Coma Scale

| Code first | Additional codes | Coding Guidelines |
|---|---|---|
| Coma in fracture of skull OR Coma in intracranial injury OR Traumatic brain injury OR Sequelae of cerebrovascular disease OR Other nontraumatic conditions, used to assess status of the central nervous system. For example, monitoring patient in intensive care unit | If available, code: R40.21 – eyes open AND R40.22 – best verbal response AND R40.23 – best motor response Add 7th character to indicate when scale was recorded*<br><br>If above measures are not available and only total score is listed- List only code R40.24- - Glasgow coma scale, total score | 7th character must be same for all R40.21-R40.23 codes<br><br>Documentation of coma scale may be based on documentation from clinicians other than physician, such as emergency medical technician. If documentation is conflicting, query the physician |

## National Institutes of Health Stroke Scale (NIHSS)

| Code first | Additional codes | Coding Guidelines |
|---|---|---|
| Acute stroke (I63) | NIHSS stroke scale (R29.7-)<br><br>Used to identify patient's neurological status and severity of stroke | Documentation of NIH stroke scale may be based on documentation from clinicians other than physician, such as emergency medical technician. Diagnosis for the stroke must be documented by patients' provider. If there is conflicting documentation, query the provider. May be recorded more than once during hospitalization |

# Coding Sepsis/Severe Sepsis

| Reason for admission | Definition | Guidelines |
|---|---|---|
| **Sepsis/Severe Sepsis Due to Infectious Process** | | |
| Sepsis due to infection | Sepsis but not severe sepsis | List code for infection<br>Do **NOT** list code from R65 category |
| Sepsis associated with organ dysfunction | Code as severe sepsis | List first code for infection<br>Then list code from R65.2- category<br>Then list code for organ dysfunction |
| Severe sepsis and organ dysfunction, not documented as related | Organ dysfunction may or may not be due to sepsis | Query provider |
| Severe sepsis and organ dysfunction, documented as related | Severe sepsis due to systemic infection with acute organ dysfunction | List first code for underlying infection<br>Then list code R65.2-<br>Then list associated organ dysfunction & localized infection if present |
| Septic shock | Cardiovascular system failure. Code as severe sepsis | List first underlying infection<br>Then list code R65.21<br>Then list code for associated organ dysfunction |
| Patient admitted with severe sepsis with localized infection | Both severe sepsis and localized infection documented at time of admission | List first code for systemic infection<br>Then list code for localized infection<br>Then list code R65.2- |
| Patient admitted with localized infection. Develops into severe sepsis after admission | Localized infection spreads to other areas during hospitalization | List first localized infection<br>Then list code for systemic infection<br>Then list code R65.2- |
| Postprocedural severe sepsis | Systemic infection following a surgical procedure | List first complication code (such as T80.2-, T81.4-, T88.0-, T86. 0-)<br>Then list code for systemic infection<br>Then list code R65.2-<br>Then list codes for any organ dysfunction |
| **Sepsis Due to Non-infectious Process** | | |
| Sepsis due to **non-infectious** process (SIRS) | Trauma, neoplasm, pancreatitis, burn or other injury. May lead to systemic infection | Circumstances of admission determine which code is listed first (non-infectious process or infection if documented)<br>Then list code R65.1-<br>Then list code for organ dysfunction |

# Guidelines for Other Specific Conditions

| Code | | Definition | Coding Guidelines |
|---|---|---|---|
| R53.2 | Functional quadriplegia | Patient unable to use limbs or ambulate (move freely) due to extreme debility (weakness). | Condition must be specifically documented as functional quadriplegia<br>Do **NOT** list this code if condition is documented as:<br>1) Neurological deficit or injury<br>2) Neurologic quadriplegia |
| R29.6 | Repeated falls | Patient has recently fallen and is now being seen to investigate reason for falls | Can be listed with Z91.81 if appropriate |
| Z91.81 | History of falls | Patient has history of falling and is at risk for falling again | Can be listed with R29.6 if appropriate |
| R99 | Death NOS | Used in very limited circumstances. Patient who has already died is brought into emergency department or other healthcare facility and is pronounced dead upon arrival | Do **NOT** list for discharge disposition of death (patient died during hospitalization) |

# Chapter 19

# Injury, Poisoning, and Certain Other
# Consequences of External Causes

These tables are taken from the Official Coding Guidelines: I.B.10 (General Coding Guidelines, Sequela [Late effects]); I.C.1.d (Certain Infectious and Parasitic Diseases, Sepsis, Severe Sepsis, and Septic Shock); I.C.2.r (Neoplasms, Malignant Neoplasm Associated with Transplanted Organs); I.C.15.r (Pregnancy, Childbirth and the Puerperium, Abuse in a Pregnant Patient); I.C.19 (Injury, Poisoning and Certain Other Consequences of External Causes); and I.C.21.c.3) (Factors Influencing Health Status and Contact with Health Services, Status).

Included in this chapter are these tables:

1) General Injury Coding Guidelines
    a. Injury Guidelines
    b. Injury Codes digits
    c. Injury Coding – 7th digits
2) Fracture coding
    a. Fracture Coding Guidelines
    b. Fracture Codes Digits
3) Burns/Corrosions Coding
    a. Burns/Corrosion Coding Guidelines
    b. Classification of Current Burns/Corrosions
4) Classification of Current Burns/Corrosions
5) Adult and Child Abuse Coding
6) Frostbite Coding
7) Complications of Care Coding
8) Poisoning, Adverse Effects, Underdosing and Toxic Effects
    a. Coding Guidelines for Poisoning, Adverse Effects, Underdosing and Toxic Effects
    b. Sequencing Codes for Poisoning, Adverse Effects, Underdosing and Toxic Effects

# General Injury Coding Guidelines

| Circumstances | Guidelines |
|---|---|
| Use of traumatic injury codes | Do **NOT** list for healing surgical wounds or complications of surgical wounds |
| Code also notes | Many codes in this chapter state: code also open wound, infection, associated fracture, etc.<br>Sequencing will depend on circumstances of admission |
| Aftercare of treatment of injury or poisoning | List injury or poisoning code with 7$^{th}$ digit for subsequent encounter<br>Do **NOT** list Z codes (aftercare) codes if 7$^{th}$ digit available |
| Complication of treatment of injury or poisoning | List first code for complication<br>Then list original injury with 7$^{th}$ digit S |
| Sepsis due to trauma, burn or other injury (SIRS) | Sequencing depends on reason for admission.<br>List first trauma, burn or other injury OR resulting systemic infection as appropriate.<br>Then list code R65.1-<br>Then list code for organ dysfunction if appropriate |
| Injury or open wound with cellulitis (acute inflammation of tissue with swelling, redness and tenderness) | List codes for both cellulitis and injury.<br>Sequencing depends on circumstances of visit<br>Code for infectious agent if applicable (B96-B96) |
| **Multiple Injuries** | |
| Primary injury results in minor damage to peripheral nerves or blood cells | List first primary injury<br>Then list codes for injury to nerves or blood vessels |
| Primary injury is blood vessels or nerves | List first injury to blood vessels or nerves<br>Then list codes for other injuries |
| Multiple injuries at different sites | Code most serious injury first (as documented by provider)<br>UNLESS a multiple site code is available (such as S30.840 – lower back and pelvis)<br>Do **NOT** list T07 (unspecified multiple injuries) unless documentation is not specific enough to select another code. |
| Superficial injuries (abrasions, contusions) and more severe injuries <u>at same site</u> | Code only the most severe injury |
| Superficial injuries (abrasions, contusion) and other injuries at <u>different sites</u> | Code all injuries documented. Code most serious injury first (as documented by provider) |

# Injury Codes Digits

| Digit | Definition | Examples |
|---|---|---|
| 1 | Injury code | S or T |
| 2 | Location of injury | Head, neck, elbow and forearm |
| 3 | Type of injury | Open wound, fracture, crushing injury |
| 4-6 | More specific information | Location, type of injury, laterality |
| 7 | Encounter | Initial encounter, subsequent encounter, sequela |

## Injury Coding – 7th Digits*

| Digits | Encounter | Definition | Examples and Guidelines |
|--------|-----------|------------|-------------------------|
| A-C | Initial encounter | Patient is receiving active treatment for the condition. | Surgical treatment<br>ER encounter<br>Evaluation and continuing treatment by new physician |
| D-R | Subsequent encounter | Active treatment has been completed.<br>Patient is seen during healing or recover phase. | Cast change or removal<br>Removal of external or internal fixation device<br>X-ray to check status of fracture<br>Medication adjustment<br>Other aftercare |
| S | Sequelae | Patient is seen for treatment of complication or conditions that arose as a direct result of the condition. | Scar formation after a burn |

*Not all injury codes include all digits A-S

7th character is determined by whether patient is receiving active treatment, not whether the provider is seeing patient for the first time.

# Fracture Coding Guidelines

| Documentation | Guidelines |
|---|---|
| Fracture not documented as open or closed | List code for closed |
| Fracture not documented as displaced or nondisplaced | List code for displaced |
| Fracture due to disease (such as bone cancer, osteoporosis, osteomalacia) | List code from chapter 13 (musculoskeletal system), NOT chapter 19 (injuries) |
| Fracture not previously treated Patient seen with fracture or malunion | List fracture code with 7$^{th}$ digit for initial encounter (A-C) |
| Fracture previously received active treatment. Patient returns with complication of fracture such as malunion or nonunion | List fracture code with 7$^{th}$ digit for subsequent care with nonunion (K, M, N) or malunion (P, Q, R) |
| Multiple fractures | List first most severe fracture Then list codes for other fractures |
| Fracture documented as open but type of fracture (I, II, IIA, etc.) not specified | Use 7$^{th}$ digit for type I or II (B, E, H. M. or Q) |

# Fracture Codes Digits

| 7$^{th}$ digit | Open or closed | Type | Healing status |
|---|---|---|---|
| 7$^{th}$ Digits for Initial encounters | | | |
| A | Closed | Not specified | Active treatment |
| B | Open | Type I or II or unspecified | Active treatment |
| C | Open | Type IIIA, IIIB or IIIC | Active treatment |
| 7$^{th}$ Digits for Subsequent encounters | | | |
| D | Closed or Unspecified | Not specified | Routine |
| E | Open | Type I or II with routine healing or unspecified | Routine |
| F | Open | Type IIIA, IIB or IIIC | Routine |
| G | Closed or Unspecified | Not specified | Delayed |
| H | Open | Type I or II or unspecified | Delayed |
| J | Open | Type IIIA, IIIB or IIIC | Delayed |
| K | Closed or Unspecified | Not specified | Nonunion |
| M | Open | Type I or II or unspecified | Nonunion |
| N | Open | Type IIIA, IIIB or IIIC | Nonunion |
| P | Closed or Unspecified | Not specified | Malunion |
| Q | Open | Type I or II or unspecified | Malunion |
| R | Open | Type IIIA, IIIB, or IIIC | Malunion |
| 7$^{th}$ Digit for Sequelae | | | |
| S | Not specified | Not specified | Healed with complication |

Note that not all fracture codes include options for all 7$^{th}$ digits listed above

# Burns/Corrosions Coding Guidelines

| Condition | Guidelines |
|---|---|
| Burns | Defined as thermal burns due to heat source, including electricity and radiation<br>Does not include sunburns. Code sunburns to category L55-<br>List also external cause codes as appropriate |
| Corrosions | Defined as burns due to chemicals<br>List additional code for poisoning or toxic effects<br>List also external cause codes as appropriate |
| First, second or third degree burns/corrosions | Most codes include digits for degrees.<br>Exception – codes for eye and internal organs |
| Nonhealing burns/ corrosions | Code as acute burn/corrosion (7th digit A) |
| Necrosis of burned skin | Code as acute burn/corrosion (7th digit A) |
| Infected burn/corrosion | List first code for burn/corrosion<br>Then list code for infection |
| Extent of body surface (T31-T32) | Listed when site is unspecified or code provides additional data<br>4th digit – Total body surface burned<br>5th digit – Percent of body surface that is 3rd degree burn |
| Burns/corrosions with other related conditions | Code all injuries<br>Sequencing depends on circumstances of admission |
| Burns/corrosions with cellulitis (acute inflammation of tissue with swelling, redness and tenderness) | List codes for both burn/corrosion and cellulitis.<br>Sequencing depends on circumstances of visit |
| Burns/corrosions with External Cause codes | List external cause codes for source, intent, and place of occurrence of burn |
| **Multiple Burns** | |
| Multiple burns/ corrosions at same site | List only one code for highest degree at that site |
| Multiple burns/ corrosions at different sites | List first code for highest degree<br>Then list codes for other burns/corrosions |
| Internal and external burns/corrosions | List codes for all burns/corrosions<br>Sequencing depends on circumstances of visit |
| **Sequelae** | |
| Sequelae of burn/corrosion | Late effects of burns/corrosions such as scar<br>List original burn/corrosion code with 7th digit S<br>In some circumstances, sequelae and current or healing burns/corrosions may be present at the same encounter. In this case:<br>1. An acute burn/corrosion (7th digit A) may be listed with sequela of burn/corrosion (7th digit D)<br>2. A healing burn/corrosion (7th digit S) may be listed with sequela of burn/corrosion (7th digit D) |

# Classification of Current Burns/Corrosions

| Degree | Definition |
|--------|------------|
| First | Erythema |
| Second | Blistering |
| Third | Full-thickness involvement |

# Adult and Child Abuse Coding

| Condition | Coding Guidelines |
|-----------|-------------------|
| Confirmed adult or child abuse | Must be documented as confirmed by provider<br>List first code T74-<br>Then list any mental health or injury codes<br>Then list external cause code for assault (X92-Y08)<br>Then list code for perpetrator of the abuse if known (Y07) |
| Suspected adult or child abuse | List first code T76-<br>Then list any mental health or injury codes<br>Do **NOT** list external cause codes |
| Suspected abuse, ruled out | List first code Z04.71 or Z04.72<br>Do **NOT** list code from categories T74 or T76<br>Do **NOT** list external cause codes |

# Frostbite Coding

| Condition | Description |
|-----------|-------------|
| Superficial frostbite | Reddened skin that turns white or pale<br>Some ice crystals may form in tissue<br>List code for hypothermia if appropriate (T68-)<br>List additional codes for external cause to indicate source, intent and place of occurrence of frostbite |
| Frostbite with tissue necrosis | Skin turns black and hard as tissue dies<br>List code for hypothermia if appropriate (T68-)<br>List additional codes for external cause to indicate source, intent and place of occurrence of frostbite |
| Frostbite with cellulitis | List codes for both frostbite and cellulitis.<br>Sequencing depends on circumstances of visit |

# Complications of Care

| Condition/Circumstances | Coding Guidelines |
|---|---|
| **General Guidelines** ||
| Intraoperative/postprocedural complications RELATED to a specific body system | Must be documented as due to procedure<br>List first code for specific complication from body system chapter |
| Intraoperative/postprocedural complications NOT related to a specific body system or involving multiple body systems | Must be documented as due to procedure<br>List code for specific complication from chapter 19 |
| Condition that MAY OR MAY NOT be related to previous procedure | Query provider |
| Pain due to medical device | List first T code<br>Then list code G89.18 or G89.28 |
| Complications with external cause codes | Some complication codes include external cause information.<br>Example - Code T81.503- – complication due to vaccination.<br>Do **NOT** list code Y69 (misadventure during medical care)<br><br>If complication code does **NOT** include external cause, list separate external cause code. |
| **Complications of Kidney Transplants** ||
| Post-transplant patient has chronic kidney disease NOT related to transplant | List Category N18 code for stage of kidney disease<br>Then list history of kidney transplant code (Z94.0) |
| Post-transplant patient has chronic kidney transplant RELATED to transplant | Condition must be documented as due to complication of transplant<br>List first code T86.1- (complication of kidney transplant)<br>Then list code for specific complication |
| **Complications of Other Transplants** ||
| Complications and rejections due to transplants<br>Condition affects function of transplanted organ | List first code from category T86-<br>Then list code for specific complication<br>Do **NOT** list code for history of transplant (Z94-) |
| Pre-existing condition or conditions that develop <u>after</u> transplant procedure ||
| Condition does NOT affect function of transplanted organ | Do **NOT** code as complication<br>List code for condition<br>Then list history of transplant code (Z94-) |
| Condition affects function of transplanted organ | List first code from category T86-<br>Then code for complication<br>Do **NOT** list code for history of transplant (Z94-) |

# Coding Guidelines for Poisoning, Adverse Effects,

## Underdosing and Toxic Effects

| Condition/Circumstances | Coding Guidelines |
|---|---|
| External cause codes | Do **NOT** list with codes for poisoning, adverse effect, underdosing and toxic effects |
| One drug/toxic substance caused more than one adverse effect, poisoning, toxic effect, or underdosing | List drug/toxic substance code only once. Example: One drug results in both fatigue and headache List code for drug once and codes for fatigue and headache |
| Two or more drugs, medicinal or biological substances involved | List code for each drug unless combination is available For example: a combination code exists for drugs related to electrolytes, caloric and water-balance agents (T50.3-) |

# Sequencing Codes for Poisoning, Adverse Effects,

## Underdosing and Toxic Effects

| Diagnosis | Definitions | Principal Diagnosis | Additional Diagnoses |
|---|---|---|---|
| Poisoning | 1. Medication not given or taken as prescribed (intentional overdose, wrong substance, wrong route of administration) 2. A prescribed drug (correctly prescribed and administered) taken with a non-prescribed drug. The two drugs interact 3. Drug interacts with alcohol 4. Overdose from use of illegal drugs | Poisoning – T36-T50 Fifth or sixth digit 1-4 to indicate intent If intent unknown, code as accidental | Condition resulting from poisoning Code for abuse or dependence of drug if applicable Condition for which drug prescribed |
| Adverse Effect | 1. Prescribed drug (correctly prescribed and administered) results in adverse effect 2. Two prescribed drugs (correctly administered) taken. The two drugs interact | Condition resulting from adverse effect | Adverse effect – T36-T50 Fifth or sixth digit 5 Condition for which drug prescribed |
| Underdosing | Patient took less of a medication than prescribed amount or manufacturer's instructions | Any relapse or exacerbation due to underdosing | Underdosing – T36-T50 Fifth or sixth digit 6 If appropriate: 1) Noncompliance (Z91.1-) 2) Complication of care (Y63-) 3) Condition for which drug prescribed |
| Toxic Effects | Harmful nonmedicinal substance is ingested or came in contact with patient | Toxic effect – T51-T65 Fifth or sixth digit 1-4 to indicate intent | Condition resulting from ingesting or having contact with toxic substance |

# Chapter 20

## External Causes of Morbidity

These tables are taken from the Official Coding Guidelines: I.B.10 (General Coding Guidelines, Sequela [Late Effects]); I.C.19 (Injury, Poisoning and Certain Other Consequences of External Causes); and I.C.20 (External Causes of Morbidity).

Included in this chapter are these tables:

1) General External Cause Coding Guidelines
2) Examples: Subsequent Visit or Sequela?
3) Coding External Causes of Injuries
4) Coding External Causes for Specific Circumstances
5) External Cause Index Entries

# General External Cause Coding Guidelines

| Circumstances | Coding Guidelines |
|---|---|
| Use of codes | Not required nationally<br>May be required by state or a specific payer<br>Never listed first |
| Use with other codes | May be listed with any code A00.9-T88.9, Z00-Z99<br>Most often listed with injury codes |
| Digits | Most codes have $7^{th}$ digits. Many codes will require X placeholders |
| Multiple external cause codes | List as many codes as needed to fully describe circumstances.<br>Claim form may limit number of codes that can be reported. If so, then -<br>List external cause codes in this order:<br>1) Code related to most serious injury due to assault, accident or self-harm<br>2) Child and adult abuse<br>3) Terrorism<br>4) Cataclysmic events (earthquake, tsunami, hurricane, etc.)<br>5) Transport accidents<br>6) Activity and external cause status<br>If multiple injuries, list first external cause code for most serious injury |
| Combination external cause codes | Codes that report sequential events such as a fall through glass with resulting striking against an object<br>Injury does not need to be specifically linked to one event or the other (the fall or the striking) regardless of which injury is more severe |
| Two or more events cause separate injuries | List external cause code for each event |
| Unknown or undetermined intent | Code as accidental.<br>All transport accidents are assumed accidental intent<br>Use undetermined only if documentation states intent cannot be determined |
| Sequelae | Late effect resulting from previous injury. Use $7^{th}$ character S on codes for original injury and external cause code but NOT on current condition (sequelae)<br>List these codes for subsequent visits for treatment of late effect of initial injury<br>Do **NOT** list sequela codes for follow-up visits if no late effect is documented<br>Do **NOT** list external cause for sequelae with external cause for related current injury |

# Examples: Subsequent Visit or Sequela?

| Subsequent Visit (Injury is healing) | Sequela (Treatment of Injury has been completed) |
|---|---|
| Delayed healing | Joint stiffness |
| Malunion | Traumatic arthritis |
| Nonunion | Contractures |

# Coding External Causes for Injuries

| Circumstances | | Codes | When Code is Used | When Code is *NOT* Used |
|---|---|---|---|---|
| **Use ALPHABETIC Index** | | | | |
| Injury | | A00-T88, Z00-Z99 | List before external cause codes | |
| **Use EXTERNAL CAUSE Index** | | | | |
| **External Cause Codes listed throughout treatment** | | | | |
| Intent and Cause of Injury | | | List before other external cause codes<br><br>If more than one cause, list code for each | Poisonings, adverse effects, underdosing or toxic effects |
| | Accidental | V00-X58 | | |
| | Intentional self-harm | X71-X83 | | |
| | Assault | X92-Y08 | | |
| | Legal intervention | Y35 | | |
| | Operations of war | Y36 | | |
| | Military operations | Y37 | | |
| | Terrorism | Y38 | Must be confirmed as terrorism by the FBI | If terrorism not confirmed by FBI, list code for assault instead |
| | Misadventures/ Complications | Y62-Y84 | Medical device malfunctions/breaks down Abnormal reaction to surgical or medical procedure | |
| **External Cause Codes listed ony for initial encounter** | | | | |
| Activity | | Y93 | List only one activity code List with cause and intent codes | Poisonings, adverse effects, under-dosing, toxic effects, misadventures, subsequent visits or sequelae Do **NOT** list Y93.9 if activity is not documented |
| Status of patient | | Y99 | List only one status code List whenever other external cause code used | Poisonings, adverse effects, under-dosing, toxic effects, misadventures, subsequent visits or sequelae If no other external cause code is being listed Do **NOT** list Y99.9 if status not documented |
| Place of occurrence | | Y92 | List only one place of occurrence code List after other external cause codes | Poisonings, adverse effects, under-dosing, toxic effects, misadventures, subsequent visits or sequelae Do **NOT** list Y92.9 if no place of occurrence documented |

External cause codes are NEVER listed as principal diangosis

For initial visit, list external cause codes in this order: Intent and cause; activity, status of patient, and place of occurrence if information is available

# Coding External Causes for Specific Circumstances

| Circumstances | Coding Guidelines |
|---|---|
| **Child or Adult Abuse** | |
| Confirmed | Must be documented as confirmed by provider<br>List first code T74-<br>Then list any mental health or injury codes<br>Then list external cause code for assault (X92-Y08)<br>Then list code for perpetrator of the abuse if known (Y07) |
| Suspected | List first code T76-<br>Then list any mental health or injury codes<br>Do **NOT** list external cause codes |
| **Terrorism** | |
| Confirmed | Must be identified as terrorism by the FBI<br>List first code for assault<br>List first code Y38 (list more than one code if more than one act of terrorism)<br>Then code for place of occurrence Y92 |
| Suspected | List code for assault<br>Do **NOT** list Y38 code |
| Secondary effects of terrorism | List first code for injury<br>List code Y38.9 for conditions occurring subsequent to terrorism event<br>Then list other Y38 codes if appropriate<br>Do **NOT** list this code for initial terrorist act |

# Using the External Cause Index

| Category of Codes | External Cause Index |
|---|---|
| Intent | Main terms:<br>Self-harm<br>Suicide<br>Assault<br>Undetermined |
| Cause of injury | Examples of Main terms and subterms:<br>Main term:  Accident<br>   caused by, due to<br>   nontraffic<br>   transport<br>       type of vehicle (such as pick-up truck,<br>        scooter, motorcyclist)<br>      Patient's role (such as driver or passenger)<br>Main term: Crushed<br>Main term: Cut<br>Main term: Contact with<br>   knife<br>   wasp |
| Activity | Examples of Main terms for activity:<br>Main terms:<br>Baseball<br>Exercise<br>Sports<br>Milking an animal |
| Place of occurrence | Main term: Place of occurrence |
| Status of patient | Main terms:<br>Status of external cause OR<br>External cause status |
| Late effects of injury | Main term: Sequela |

# Chapter 21

# Factors Influencing Health Status and

# Contact with Health Services

These tables are taken from the Official Coding Guidelines: I.C.21 (Factors Influencing Health Status and Contact with Health Services).

Included in this chapter are these tables:

1) General Coding Guidelines
2) Categories of Codes
3) Guidelines for Status, Aftercare, Follow-up Care, History and Screening Codes
4) Coding for Obstetrical and Reproductive Health Services
5) Coding for Conditions in the Newborn

## General Coding Guidelines

| | Coding Guidelines |
|---|---|
| Use of Z codes | Use in any healthcare setting<br>These are diagnosis codes. List with appropriate procedure codes. |
| Sequencing | Circumstances of encounter will determine if code listed first or as additional code<br>See list of Z codes that can only be listed first in the Coding Guidelines I.C.21.c.11). |
| Nonspecific Z codes | These include nonspecific codes and circumstances that can be coded elsewhere.<br>Inpatient setting - little reason to list these codes<br>Outpatient setting – list only when there is a need for further documentation<br>Example: Z02.9 – encounter for administrative examinations, unspecified |

## Categories of Z Codes

| Codes | Definition | Guidelines |
|---|---|---|
| Contact/Exposure Z20-, Z77 | Patient has no signs or symptoms of condition but is suspected to have been exposed to it by:<br>1) Close personal contact with infected individual OR<br>2) Having been in an area where disease is epidemic | List first if reason for encounter is testing<br>List as additional code to identify potential risk |
| Inoculations and vaccinations Z23 | Prophylactic inoculation | List with procedure codes for administration of vaccine and types of immunization given<br>List first if reason for encounter<br>List as additional code if performed during routine preventive visit (such as well-baby visit) |
| Observation Z03-Z05 | Codes used in very limited circumstances when person is being observed for a suspected condition that is ruled out | Always listed first EXCEPT for Z05 (newborn). If this is the episode of birth, code Z38 first.<br><br>List additional codes only if unrelated to suspected condition<br>Do **NOT** list when injury, illness or sign/symptom related to the suspected condition is present. List code for the condition with external cause code if appropriate |
| Counseling Z30-Z32.3, Z69-Z71, Z76.81 | Patient or family member receives assistance:<br>1) In the aftermath of an illness or injury OR<br>2) Support needed to cope with family or social problems | Do **NOT** list with diagnosis code when the counseling is considered integral to standard treatment (for example, routine annual exam) |
| Routine and administrative exams Z00-Z02 | Encounters for routine exams, general checkups or administrative exams | Always listed first except for Z00.6<br>Do **NOT** list this code if exam is done to diagnose a suspected condition<br>If condition is found during exam:<br>1) List first code for exam<br>2) Then code condition found<br>Some codes include digits to indicate whether or not abnormal findings were found during the exam. If results are not available at time of coding, list code for without abnormal findings.<br>List additional codes for pre-existing or chronic conditions IF conditions are not focus of visit |

**CONTINUED ON NEXT PAGE**

88

## Categories of Z Codes (continued)

| Codes | Definition | Guidelines |
|---|---|---|
| Laboratory exams - Z01.8- | Encounters for pre-operative and pre-procedural laboratory exams | Always listed first<br>Do **NOT** list code:<br>1) With codes for administrative exams<br>2) For exams related to pregnancy and reproduction |
| Donation of organ or tissue – Z52 | Living individual seen for donation of blood or other body tissue | Always listed first except for code Z52.9<br>Do **NOT** list code if:<br>1) Self-donation (such as harvesting of patient's skin for use by patient)<br>2) Donation is from cadavers |
| Prophylactic organ removal - Z40- | Normal tissue (organ) is removed due to genetic susceptibility or family history of malignancy<br>Done as preventative measure | List first code Z40-<br>Then list code for susceptibility or family history if appropriate<br>If patient had malignancy of one site and is having prophylactic removal at another site to prevent new malignancy or metastatic disease – code first Z40.0 and then malignancy code<br>Do **NOT** list code Z40.0 if patient is having organ removal for treatment of malignancy (not prophylactic) |

# Guidelines for Status, Aftercare, Follow-up Care, History and Screening Codes

| Code/Circumstance | Definition | Coding Guidelines |
|---|---|---|
| Status | Patient is carrier of a disease or has sequelae or residual of past disease or condition<br>Examples: presence of prosthetic device, sterilization status | Do **NOT** list with code from body system chapter if both codes include same information. For example: heart transplant status (Z94.1) with complications of heart transplant (T86.2-). Code only T86.2- code |
| **Patient _STILL_ has condition** | | |
| Weaning from mechanical ventilator | Patient has been on mechanical ventilator but is now being weaned off ventilator | List first code from category J96.1-<br>Then list code Z99.11 |
| Aftercare | Continued care during healing or recovery phase or treatment of long-term consequences of disease<br><br>Examples: Fitting and adjustment of device, attention to artificial openings | Usually listed first but may be listed second if appropriate to provide additional detail:<br>1) To describe resolving condition/sequelae.<br>2) With status Z codes to indicate nature of aftercare (for example, Z95.1 {presence of bypass graft] with Z48.812 [aftercare for surgery on circulatory system}]). If one code incudes sufficient information, list only one code (for example, Z43.0, encounter for attention to tracheostomy.)<br>Do **NOT** list for:<br>1) Current, acute disease. Exceptions are Z51.0 and Z51.1<br>2) Aftercare of injury. Use 7th digit S on injury code |
| **Patient had condition in the past but it _NO LONGER_ exists at time of encounter** | | |
| Personal history | Patient's past medical condition that:<br>1) No longer exists<br>2) Is not receiving any treatment<br>3) Has the potential for recurrence and<br>4) Requires continued monitoring. | May be listed:<br>1) With follow-up codes. List follow-up code first<br>2) With any other codes regardless of reason for visit |
| Follow-up Z08, Z09, Z39 | Patient seen for continuing surveillance following completed treatment of a disease, condition or injury. | May be listed:<br>1) With history codes. List follow-up code first<br>2) To explain multiple visits.<br>Do **NOT** list if condition is found to have recurred during follow-up visit. List diagnosis code instead |
| **Patient NEVER had the condition or signs or symptoms of it** | | |
| Screening | Testing for disease or disease precursors in seemingly well individuals so that early detection and treatment can be provided | List first if reason for visit is the screening. List as additional code if patient seen for other condition and screening also done. .<br>If condition found during screening, list first screening code, then code for condition<br>Do **NOT** list screening code if:<br>1) Screening is part of routine exam (For example, pap smear during routine gyn exam)<br>2) Patient has signs or symptoms of condition. List code for diagnostic exam |
| Family history | Patient has family member(s) who has had a disease; patient is considered at higher risk of also contracting the disease. | May be listed with:<br>1) Screening codes to explain reason for screening<br>2) Any other codes regardless of reason for visit |

# Coding for Obstetrical and Reproductive Health Services

| Code | | Coding Guidelines |
|---|---|---|
| Z03.7- | Encounter for suspected maternal and fetal conditions ruled out | Always listed first.<br>List additional codes only if reporting conditions unrelated to suspected condition.<br>Do **NOT** list this code:<br>1)   If condition is confirmed or signs/symptoms are documented.<br>2)   For encounters for antenatal screening. See code Z36 |
| | Observation and testing for abnormal condition in fetus. Test results are not definitive | List code for O35, O36, O40, or O41<br>Do **NOT** list observation codes Z03-Z04 |
| Z30 | Encounter for contraceptive management | Patient is trying **NOT** to become pregnant |
| Z31 | Encounter for procreative management | Patient is trying to become pregnant |
| Z32.0- | Encounter for pregnancy test | 5$^{th}$ digit indicates results - unknown, positive or negative |
| Z32.2 | Encounter for childbirth instruction | |
| Z32.3 | Encounter for childcare instruction | |
| Z33.1 | Pregnancy incidental | Patient seen for condition documented as unrelated to pregnancy<br>List first unrelated condition<br>Then list this code |
| Z33.2 | Encounter for elective termination of pregnancy | Always listed first<br>Then list codes from chapter 15 if appropriate<br>Code listed when termination was uncomplicated<br>Do **NOT** list this code with codes for complications of abortion |
| Z34- | Encounter for supervision of normal pregnancy | Always listed first<br>Code listed for routine antepartum visit without complications<br>Do **NOT** list with any codes from chapter 15 |
| Z36 | Encounter for antenatal screening of mother | List for routine screening<br>Mother and fetus have no signs or symptoms of abnormal condition |
| Z3A | Weeks of gestation | Never listed first<br>List on maternal record<br>If complication present at admission, list code for weeks for date of admission<br>If complication develops after admission, list code for weeks for when complication developed<br>Do NOT use this code for pregnancies with abortive outcomes, elective termination of pregnancy, or for postpartum conditions |
| Z37 | Outcome of delivery | Never listed first<br>List on maternal record when delivery occurred during this admission<br>Do **NOT** list on newborn record |
| Z76.81 | Counseling for expectant mother | List for prebirth visit with potential pediatrician |

## Coding for Conditions in the Newborn

| Code | | Coding Guidelines |
|---|---|---|
| Z00.1- | Encounter for routine child health exam | Always listed first<br>Child is under 29 days old<br>If abnormal findings during exam:<br>List first Z00.1- code<br>Then list code for any findings |
| Z38- | Liveborn infants according to place of birth and type of delivery | Always listed first on newborn record<br>Do **NOT** list on maternal record |
| Z76.1- | Encounter for health supervision and care of foundling (baby that has been abandoned) | Always listed first |

BranTLEY

Made in the USA
Middletown, DE
15 November 2016